101

blender drinks

Special thanks to Vita-Mix and my "Book Club" focus group. All of you were a great help.

This book is printed on acid-free paper.

Copyright © 2010 by Kim Haasarud. All rights reserved.

Photography copyright © 2010 by Alexandra Grablewski

Food styling by Brian Preston-Campbell

Prop styling by Leslie Siegel

Published by John Wiley & Sons, Inc., Hoboken, New Jersey

Published simultaneously in Canada

For general information on our other products and services or for technical support, please contact our Customer Care Department within the United States at (800) 762-2974, outside the United States at (317) 572-3993 or fax (317) 572-4002.

Wiley also publishes its books in a variety of electronic formats. Some content that appears in print may not be available in electronic books. For more information about Wiley products, visit our web site at www.wiley.com.

Library of Congress Cataloging-in-Publication Data:

Haasarud, Kim.

101 blender drinks / Kim Haasarud ; photography by Alexandra Grablewski.

p. cm.

Includes index.

ISBN 978-0-470-50513-7 (cloth)

1. Blenders (Cookery) 2. Cocktails. I. Title. II. Title: One hundred and one blender drinks.

TX840.B5H376 2010

641.8'74--dc22

2009023916

Printed in the United States of America

10 9 8 7 6

101
blender drinks

KIM HAASARUD
PHOTOGRAPHY BY ALEXANDRA GRABLEWSKI

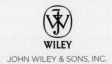

WILEY
JOHN WILEY & SONS, INC.

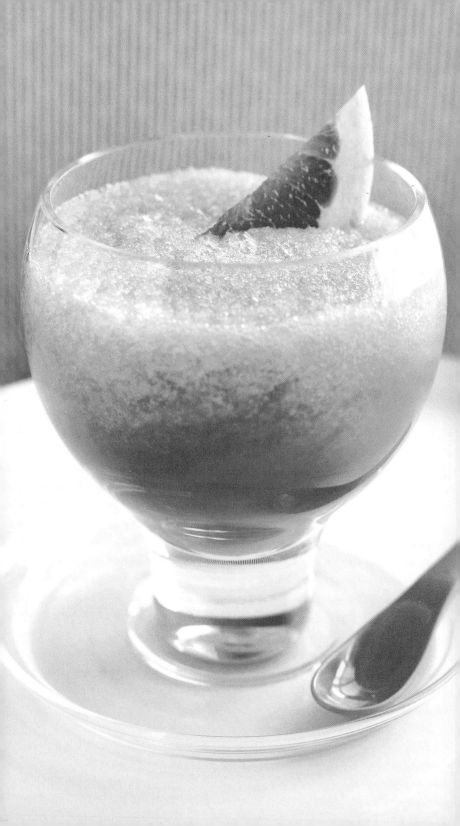

introduction

When people hear "blender drink" or "frozen drink," they most probably think of sipping a tall, cool one while sitting on a beach, or maybe a morning smoothie. But with the mixology movement happening across the United States, along with raised awareness of local ingredients, the number of various combinations for frozen drinks is limitless. Anything can be blended, from fruits to vegetables to nuts to herbs to sparkling beverages.

Throughout this book, you'll find some standard classics like the Strawberry Daiquiri, Frozen Margarita, and Piña Colada, but you'll also find unique combinations such as the Thai Colada (with ground cardamom), the Acai Margarita, Brazilian Batidas, frozen champagne cocktails like the Jasmine Peach Bellini, and frozen sangrias. I was inspired by great food chefs like Jamie Oliver, Tyler Florence, and Giada De Laurentiis and created some frozen libations around some of their dishes. I also included some recipes from some of my mixologist friends.

There are some amazing things you can do with a blender besides just blending the drink. Vitamix, one of the major manufacturers of blenders, sent me one of theirs to play around with, and I have to say, well, it was love at first sight. There are so many things you can do with it, from grinding your own spices to making specialty purees and whipped creams. You can also make your own nut milks for use not only in blended drinks but in classic cocktails as well. There are also blending "techniques" one can use that will create different textures and shapes of the ice. For example, if you blend the ingredients first and then add the ice, it makes for an extremely smooth, sometimes even frothy, drink, and the ice does not water it down. Who knew?

So, whip out the blender and get crackin'. Before you know it, you'll be singing the words of Garth Brooks: "Give me two piña coladas . . . I gotta have one for each hand!"

Cheers!

BLENDING TIPS
Tip #1: Blending with Ice

There are many types of ice, ranging from half-moons to cubes to crushed, that can be found in people's freezers or at the grocery store, and they all can greatly affect the texture of a blended drink and the amount of dilution as it melts. Even though the recipes may call for a cup or two of ice, the best way to determine how much ice you need is just to eyeball it. The first step is to blend the ingredients first *without* the ice. Then, slowly add a few cubes of ice at a time until the drink reaches the texture you want. I like my blended cocktails to be sippable, meaning that I don't have to tap the back of the glass or use a spoon to get the contents to move. The drink should easily flow out of the blender cup. If the contents immediately start to separate in the glass, you need to add more ice. If you have trouble getting the contents out of the blender cup, you used too much ice.

Tip #2: Fresh vs. Frozen

Fresh, seasonal fruit that you find at your local farmer's market is always best. But in some cases you can use frozen fruit, such as peaches, mango, berries, and so forth. I have found that the frozen fruit isn't nearly as sweet as the fresh stuff, so you many need to add a little sugar (or simple syrup) to taste.

Tip #3: Sugar

In the recipes where I call for simple syrup (see recipe on opposite page), you can also just add regular granulated sugar, Splenda, or a number of different sweeteners including agave nectar, honey, brown sugar, Demerara sugar, confectioners' sugar, sanding sugars, and so on. The blender instantly disperses them evenly. (Even some fruits can take the place of sugar, such as white grapes.)

Also note that a regular recipe on the rocks—such as a Margarita—requires more sugar if you're going to blend it. So, always keep extra on hand.

SIMPLE SYRUP

1 cup sugar
1 cup hot water

In a small bowl or glass, combine the sugar with the hot water and stir until completely dissolved. Let cool completely before using. Keep covered and refrigerated.

Tip #4: Cleaning

Always try to rinse the blender cup and base right after use. They are super-easy to clean—the ingredients rinse right off. However, if you're like me and occasionally leave the blender cup in the sink overnight (my bad), it's much more difficult to clean and can be dangerous if you try to scrub the blades. One trick I found is to put some hot soapy water in the blender cup and blend it clean! Just make sure the lid is on tight and that the water isn't scalding hot.

BLENDED EXTRAS AND SUBSTITUTIONS
Syrups

In addition to simple syrup, there are many other syrups one can use in a blended drink. Monin is a large syrup manufacturer whose products can be found in many grocery stores.

Or, you can make your own. Just use the same basic recipe as simple syrup, 1 part water to 1 part sugar. Below are a few syrup recipes that can be substituted for simple syrup. But, the possibilities are endless.

HONEY WATER

1 cup of honey (can use any type—clover, orange blossom, buckwheat, etc.)
1 cup of water

Combine the honey and water in a saucepan over medium heat. Keep stirring until the honey has completely dissolved. Keep covered and refrigerated until ready to use.

HIBISCUS ORANGE SYRUP

2 cups steeped hibiscus tea
2 cups white sugar
3 orange wheels

Combine the hibiscus tea, sugar, and orange wheels into a large pan over medium heat. Keep stirring until the mixture starts to boil. Once it starts to boil, take off the heat and let rest/cool. Strain. Keep covered and refrigerated until ready to use.

JASMINE TEA SYRUP

2 cups steeped jasmine tea
2 cups white sugar

Combine the jasmine tea with the sugar into a large pan over medium heat. Keep stirring until the mixture starts to boil. Once it starts to boil, take off the heat and let rest/cool. Strain. Keep covered and refrigerated until ready to use. Makes about 6 ounces of syrup.

Purees

Purees are super-simple to make and great for cocktails, whether frozen, on the rocks, or straight up.

BERRY PUREE

1 cup berries, rinsed
Simple syrup (see page 7), to taste

Blend the berries in the blender. Add simple syrup if needed to thin it out—you may only need a splash of it.

STONE FRUIT PUREES

Stone fruit (peaches, nectarines, apricots, plums, etc.)
Simple syrup (see page 7), to taste

Blanch the fruits in a pot of boiling water for 5 minutes. Remove from the heat and let the fruit cool. The skins should come right off. Cut into chunks and place in the blender. Add simple syrup, if needed, to help thin it out—you may only need a splash of it.

ORCHARD FRUIT PUREES

Orchard fruit (apples, pears), peeled, cored, and cut into chunks
Apple juice or pear nectar

Blend the fruit in the blender. Add the juice to help thin out—you may only need a splash of it.

Milks & Whipped Creams

In many recipes I use a light cream or milk. But for those who are lactose intolerant, try using (or making) your own nut milks with the blender.

ALMOND MILK

1 cup raw almonds
3 cups water, plus extra for soaking
Sweetener (such as agave nectar, sugar, honey, etc.; optional)
Flavoring ingredient (such as vanilla beans or extract, dates, berries, etc.; optional)

Soak the raw almonds in a bowl of water overnight in the refrigerator. Drain and rinse the almonds and place in the blender. Add the 3 cups water and blend until smooth, about 20 seconds. Strain through cheesecloth or a fine-mesh sieve. Rinse out the blender cup and pour the almond milk back into the cup. Add any other sweeteners or ingredients, if desired, and blend. Cover and keep refrigerated.

RICE MILK

4 cups water
1 cup cooked rice (white or brown)
1 vanilla bean (or ½ teaspoon vanilla extract)
Sweetener (4 tablespoons sugar or honey, to taste; optional)
Ground cinnamon (for the Mexican drink horchata; optional)

In a saucepan, combine the water, rice, vanilla bean, sweetener, if desired, and cinamon, if using, and bring to a boil. Let simmer for 10 minutes. Transfer to a blender and blend until smooth. Strain through cheesecloth or a fine-mesh sieve. Cover and keep refrigerated.

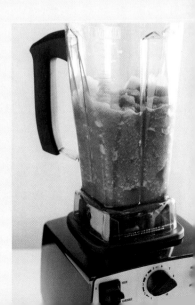

Whipped Creams

You can also make your own whipped creams as an added garnish. Simply blend heavy whipping cream in the blender on medium for 10 to 15 seconds and voilà! But be careful, for it is very easy to over-blend and get to the "butter" stage. Add different sanding sugars for different colors. You can also fold in various spirits, like sherry, or chocolate sauce for some decadent whipped creams. Below are few recipes.

SHERRY CRÈME
Great to serve on top of chocolate or coffee blended drinks.

> 1 cup heavy whipping cream
> 2 tablespoons sugar (optional)
> 1 ounce cream sherry

Pour the cream and sugar, if desired, into a blender and blend until whipped, about 10 to 15 seconds. You should be able to turn the blender cup upside down and the contents won't spill out. Scoop the contents into a bowl. Fold in the sherry.

STRAWBERRY OR BLACKBERRY TRIFLE CREAM
Great to top off frozen drinks with strawberries or even chocolate drinks.

> 1 cup heavy whipping cream
> ½ cup hulled strawberries (or 5 to 6 blackberries)
> 1 graham cracker square
> 1 tablespoon sugar
> 1 ounce cordial (such as Licor 43, Tuaca, or Grand Marnier; optional)

Combine the cream, berries, graham cracker, and sugar in a blender and blend until smooth. Do not over-blend. Fold in the liqueur, if desired.

CHOCOLATE CHIP CREAM

> 1 cup heavy whipping cream
> ¼ cup semi-sweet chocolate chips
> 1 tablespoon sugar
> ⅛ teaspoon crème de menthe or peppermint schnapps
>   (or extract; optional for a chocolate mint version)
> 1 ounce Baileys Mocha or Baileys Chocolate Mint (optional)

Combine the cream, chocolate chips, sugar, and crème de menthe in a blender. Blend for 20 seconds. Fold in the Baileys, if desired.

Ground Spices

Some recipes call for a sprinkle or dash of ground cinnamon, nut-meg, or cardamom, to name just a few spices. Nothing beats freshly ground spices versus buying them already ground. You can even do a combination of spices, for example a nutmeg-cinnamon-sugar spice. To make your own, make sure the blender cup is *completely* dry. Add the whole spices and blend until ground. It takes about 30 seconds—it will look like a mini tornado in the blender.

You can also use the ground spices to rim the cocktail glass. Simply wet the rim with a lemon wedge and dip into the ground spice.

CINNAMON-NUTMEG-SUGAR SPICE

    4 cinnamon sticks
    1 whole nutmeg
    2 tablespoons sugar

In a dry blender cup, combine the cinnamon sticks and nutmeg. Blend until completely ground. Stir in the sugar. Keep in a dry container.

CARDAMOM-SUGAR SPICE

    5 white cardamom pods
    3 tablespoons sugar

In a dry blender cup, blend the cardamom until completely ground. Stir in the sugar. Keep in a dry container.

Fresh Sour

Throughout the book, some of the recipes call for a fresh sour mix. Trust me, store-bought sweet-and-sour mix cannot even come close to making your own fresh sour. Here is a tried-and-true recipe.

    2 cups simple syrup (page 7)
    1 cup fresh lime juice (about 8 limes)
    1 cup fresh lemon juice (about 7 lemons)

Combine the ingredients in a measuring cup. Funnel into a clean, empty bottle. Keep covered and refrigerated.

1 FROZEN MARGARITA

Lime wedge and kosher salt, for garnishing rim (optional)
2 ounces pure agave tequila
1 ounce orange liqueur
1 ounce fresh lime juice
1½ ounces simple syrup (see page 7)
½ ounce fresh lemon juice
Lime wheel, for garnish

If desired, wet the outside rim of a cocktail or Margarita glass with a lime wedge. Dip into a plate of kosher salt and set aside.

Combine the tequila, orange liqueur, lime juice, simple syrup, and lemon juice in a blender with 1 cup of ice. Blend until smooth. Pour into the glass. Garnish with the lime wheel.

2 AMAZON CHERRY MARGARITA (ACAI MARGARITA)

2 ounces reposado tequila
1 ounce Cointreau
1 ounce acai juice (such as Sambazon)
1 ounce fresh lime juice
1 ounce simple syrup (see page 7)
Splash of pomegranate juice
Lime wheel, for garnish

Combine the tequila, Cointreau, acai juice, lime juice, simple syrup, and pomegranate juice in a blender with 1 cup of ice. Blend until smooth. Pour into a cocktail or Margarita glass. Garnish with the lime wheel.

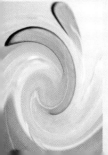

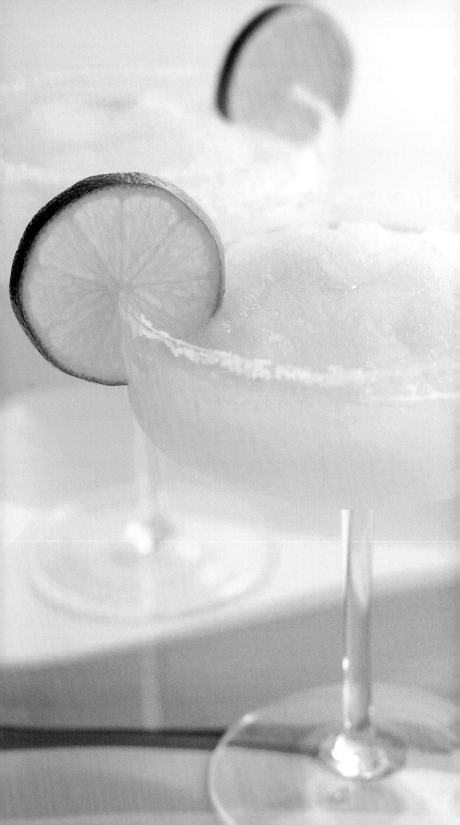

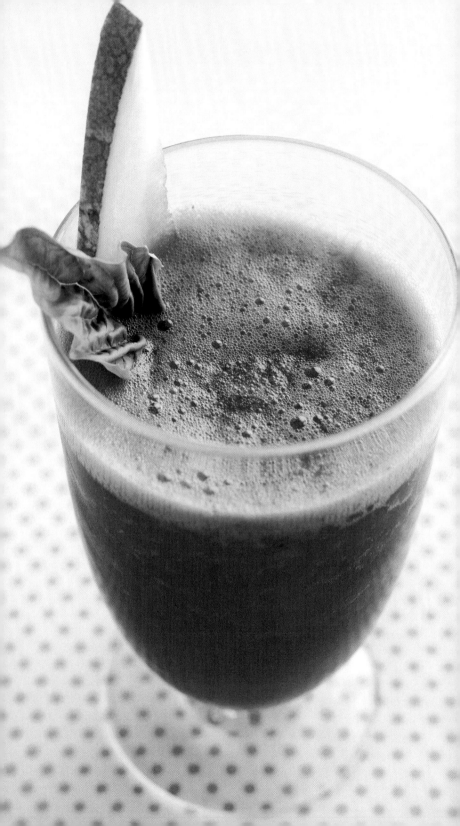

3 WATERMELON-BASIL MARGARITA

The flavor of watermelon can vary from one to the next, with some being very flavorful and juicy and others being a bit blander. I like to use watermelon schnapps just to pump up the flavor a bit, but not to act as the sole watermelon flavor.

2 ounces reposado tequila
1 ounce watermelon schnapps
1 cup fresh watermelon chunks
1 ounce fresh lime juice
1 ounce simple syrup (see page 7)
2 basil leaves
Watermelon wedge (or 3 watermelon seeds), for garnish

Combine the tequila, schnapps, watermelon chunks, lime juice, simple syrup, and 1 basil leaf in a blender with 1 cup of ice. Blend until smooth. Pour into a cocktail or Margarita glass. Garnish with the watermelon wedge and the remaining basil leaf.

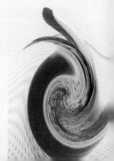

4 POMEGRANATE-GINGER MARGARITA

2 ounces silver tequila
1 ounce triple sec
1½ ounces pomegranate juice
1 ounce fresh lime juice
1 ounce simple syrup (see page 7)
½ teaspoon ginger juice (sold by the bottle at many grocery stores)
Candied ginger, for garnish

Combine the tequila, triple sec, pomegranate juice, lime juice, simple syrup, and ginger juice in a blender with 1 cup of ice. Blend until smooth. Pour into a cocktail or Margarita glass. Garnish with candied ginger.

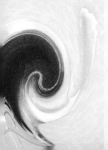

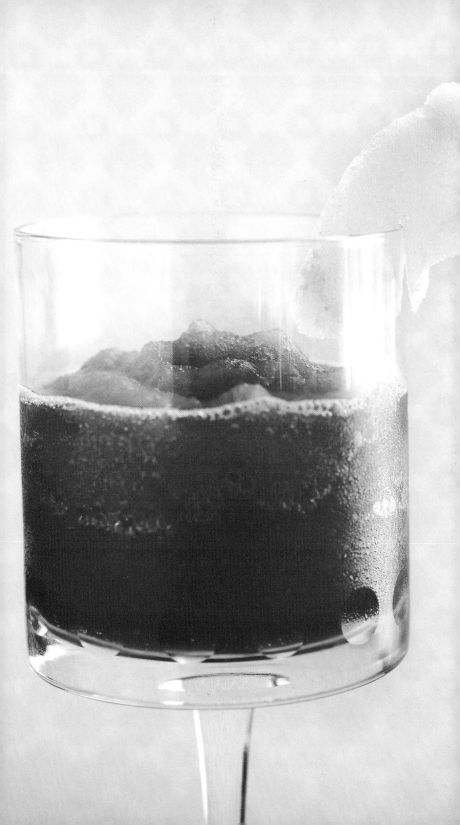

5 PAPAYA ZINGER

MAKES 2 SERVINGS

1½ cups fresh papaya chunks
½ cup fresh pineapple chunks
2 ounces reposado tequila
1 ounce triple sec
1 ounce fresh lime juice
1 ounce orange juice
½ ounce simple syrup (see page 7)
2 lemon wheels, for garnish

Combine the papaya, pineapple, tequila, triple sec, lime juice,
orange juice, and simple syrup in a blender with 1 cup of ice. Blend
until smooth. Pour into two cocktail or Margarita glasses. Garnish
each with a lemon wheel.

A NOTE ON DAIQUIRIS

The Daiquiri is one of those drinks that has been radi-
cally manipulated over the past few decades—not in a
good way—and is mostly seen coming out of a frozen
drink machine made with an overly sweet cocktail mix.
A classic Daiquiri is a simple one—rum, lime, and sugar.
I've expanded on the Daiquiri using many fresh ingredients, but the base will always remain the same.

6 PEACHY LIME DAIQUIRI

MAKES 2 SERVINGS

  1 peach (blanched, peeled, and cut into chunks)
  4 ounces light rum
  1 ounce peach liqueur
  2 ounces fresh lime juice
  2 ounces simple syrup (see page 7)
  2 lime wheels, for garnish

Combine the peach, rum, peach liqueur, lime juice, and simple
syrup in a blender with 2 cups of ice. Blend until smooth. Pour into
two cocktail glasses. Garnish each with a lime wheel.

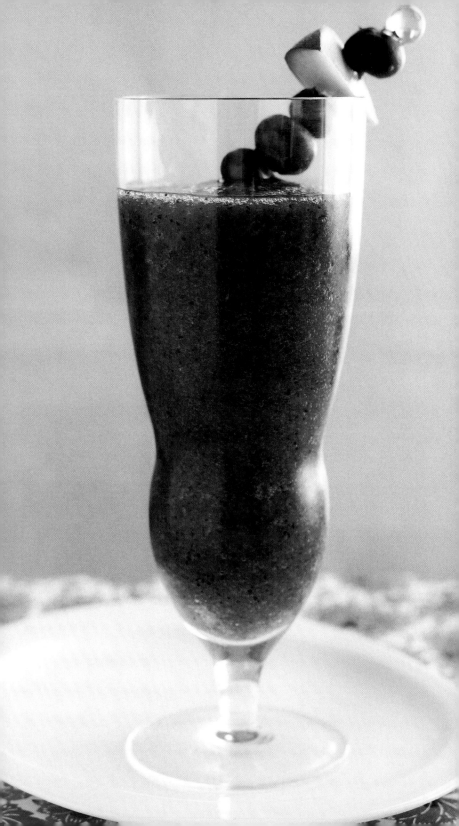

7 BLUEBERRY-PEACH DAIQUIRI

MAKES 2 SERVINGS

1 peach (blanched, peeled, and cut into chunks)
½ cup fresh blueberries
2 ounces light rum
1 ounce blueberry syrup (such as Monin)
1 ounce lime juice
½ ounce peach liqueur
2 peach wedges and 8 blueberries, for garnish

Combine the peach, blueberries, rum, blueberry syrup, lime juice, and peach liqueur in a blender with 1 cup of ice. Blend until smooth. Pour into two cocktail glasses. Garnish each with 4 skewered blueberries and 1 peach wedge.

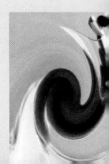

8 AT FIRST BLUSH

MAKES 2 TO 3 SERVINGS

2 ounces light rum
2 ounces simple syrup (see page 7)
1 ounce raspberry liqueur (such as Mathilde)
1 ounce rosé champagne (such as Chandon Rose)
1 ounce fresh lime juice
2 or 3 strawberries, hulled, plus 1 to 1½ for garnish
2 or 3 sage leaves, for garnish

Combine the rum, simple syrup, raspberry liqueur, rosé champagne, lime juice, and the 2 or 3 strawberries in a blender with 2 cups of ice. Blend until smooth. Pour into two or three cocktail glasses (or champagne flutes for a festive feel). Garnish each with a half strawberry and a sage leaf.

9 TAHITIAN PINEAPPLE DAIQUIRI

1½ ounces rum
1 ounce Navan vanilla liqueur
1 ounce pineapple juice
1 ounce coconut cream (such as Coco Lopez)
½ ounce fresh lime juice
Pineapple wedge, for garnish

Combine the rum, vanilla liqueur, pineapple juice, coconut cream, and lime juice in a blender with 1 cup of ice. Blend until smooth. Pour into a cocktail glass. Garnish with the pineapple wedge.

10 STRAWBERRY-BANANA DAIQUIRI

4 strawberries, hulled, plus 1 for garnish
½ banana, peeled plus 1 chunk for garnish
2 ounces rum
1½ ounces fresh lime juice
2 ounces simple syrup (see page 7)

Combine the 4 strawberries, ½ banana, rum, lime juice, and simple syrup in a blender with a half cup of ice. Blend until smooth. Pour into a cocktail glass. Garnish with the remaining strawberry and the banana chunk.

BATIDAS

Batidas are the classic cocktails of Brazil, consisting of blended fruits, cachaça (Brazilian rum), and some-times condensed milk (or "table cream"). They are delicious—come up with your own version using any sort of fresh seasonal fruits.

11 MANGO BATIDA

1 cup fresh mango chunks, plus 1 slice for garnish
2 ounces cachaça
2 ounces sweetened condensed milk
Splash of coconut milk

Combine the mango chunks, cachaça, condensed milk, and coconut milk in a blender on high for 10 seconds. Add 1 cup of crushed ice and blend for 3 seconds. Pour into a rocks glass and garnish with the mango slice.

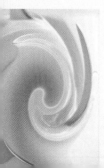

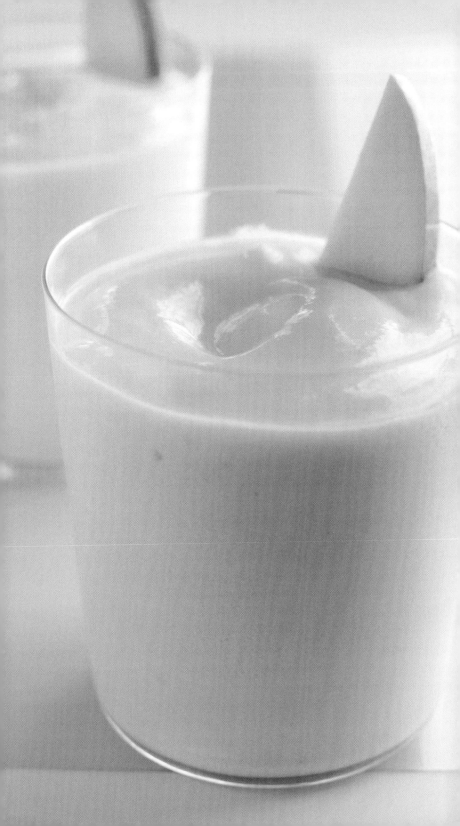

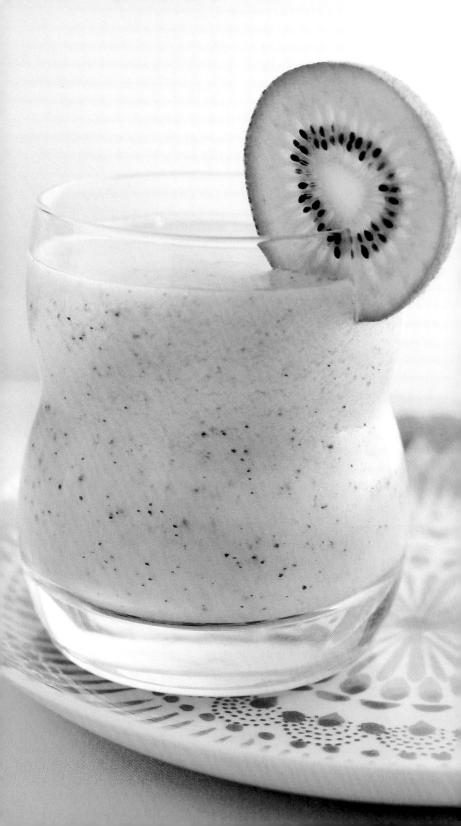

12 KIWI-COCO BATIDA

2 ounces cachaça
1 whole kiwi, peeled and cut into chunks (reserve 1 slice for garnish)
1 ounce coconut syrup
1 ounce sweetened condensed milk
Splash of coconut milk

Combine the cachaça, kiwi, coconut syrup, condensed milk, and coconut milk in a blender on high for 10 seconds. Add 1 cup of crushed ice and blend for 3 seconds. Pour into a rocks glass and garnish with the kiwi slice.

13 BLUEBERRY BATIDA

2 ounces cachaça
1 ounce sweetened condensed milk
10 to 15 blueberries, a few reserved for garnish
½ ounce blueberry syrup

Combine the cachaça, condensed milk, blueberries, and blueberry syrup in a blender on high for 10 seconds. Add 1 cup of crushed ice and blend for 3 seconds. Pour into a rocks glass and garnish with the reserved blueberries.

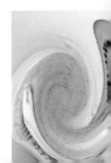

14 BRAZILIAN PEPPER CRUSH

2 ounces cachaça
2 ounces fresh sour (see page 11)
1 tablespoon jalapeño-orange marmalade (or other marmalade
  or jam with jalapeños)
2 kumquats
Splash of grenadine
1 fresh jalapeño, sliced, for garnish (optional)

Combine the cachaça, fresh sour, marmalade, 1 of the kumquats,
and grenadine in a blender on high for 10 seconds. Add 5 to 7 ice
cubes and blend until smooth. Pour into a rocks glass. Garnish with
the sliced jalapeño and the remaining kumquat.

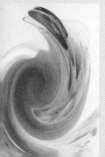

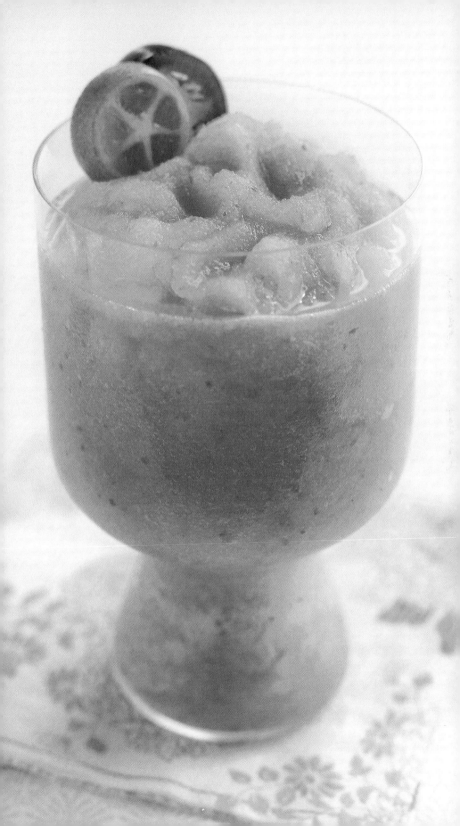

15 FROZEN LEMONADE

3 ounces fresh lemon juice
4 ounces simple syrup (see page 7)
1½ ounces citrus vodka (optional)
½ teaspoon lemon zest (optional)
Lemon wheel, for garnish

Combine the lemon juice, simple syrup, vodka, if desired, and lemon zest, if desired, in a blender with 1 cup of ice. Blend until smooth. Pour into a cocktail glass. Garnish with the lemon wheel.

16 FROZEN LIMEADE

3 ounces fresh lime juice
4 ounces simple syrup (see page 7)
1½ ounces citrus vodka or light rum
Lime wheel, for garnish

Combine the lime juice, simple syrup, and vodka in a blender with 1 cup of ice. Blend until smooth. Pour into a cocktail glass. Garnish with the lime wheel.

17 KIWI-MELON KRUSH

MAKES 2 SERVINGS

1½ cups fresh honeydew melon
1 whole kiwi, peeled
2 ounces Midori
2 ounces orange juice, plus extra if needed
2 small melon wedges and 2 kiwi slices, for garnish

Combine the melon, kiwi, Midori, and orange juice in a blender
with 1 cup of ice. Blend until smooth and add more orange juice, if
needed. Pour into two cocktail (or juice) glasses. Garnish each with
a melon wedge and a kiwi slice.

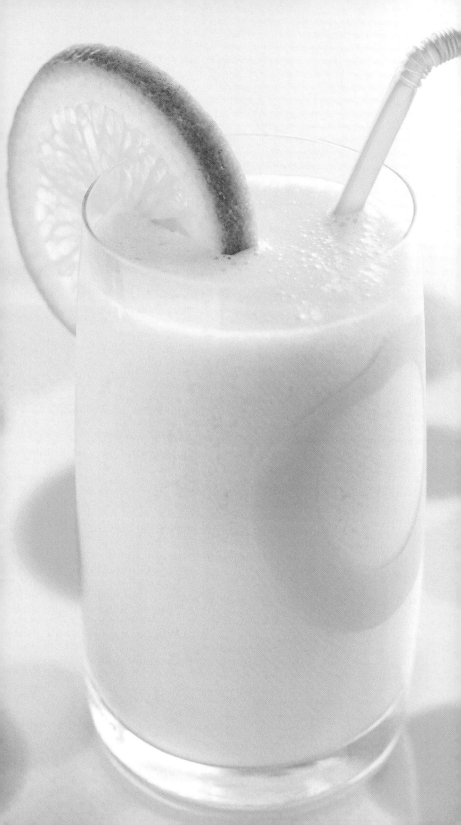

18 ORANGE JULIUS MAXIMUS

MAKES 2 SERVINGS

Just like the classic, but with an alcoholic punch. As much as I am
a fan of freshly squeezed juices, this drink really needs the concentrate versus the fresh.

1½ cups half-and-half
4 ounces simple syrup (see page 7)
2 ounces orange juice concentrate
2 ounces vanilla vodka
2 orange wheels, for garnish

Combine the half-and-half, simple syrup, orange juice concentrate,
and vodka in a blender with a few ice cubes. Blend until smooth
and add more ice, if necessary. Pour into two juice glasses and garnish each with an orange wheel.

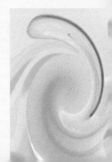

19 GUAVA LAVA PASSION

1 ounce raspberry puree
1½ ounces fresh lime juice
2 ounces simple syrup (see page 7)
1½ ounces mango rum
½ ounce guava puree
½ ounce passion fruit puree
Lime wedge and raspberry, for garnish

In the bottom of a Hurricane glass or other large glass, pour in the raspberry puree; set aside. Combine the lime juice, simple syrup, mango rum, guava puree, and passion fruit puree in a blender with 1 cup of ice. Blend until smooth. Pour into the glass. Garnish with a lime wedge and a raspberry.

20 PAPAYA-ORANGE CRUSH

½ cup fresh papaya chunks
4 ounces orange juice
1½ ounces orange vodka
Simple syrup (see page 7), to taste, if needed
Sage sprig and lime wedge, for garnish

Combine the papaya, orange juice, vodka, and simple syrup, if using, in a blender with 1 cup of ice. Blend until smooth. Pour into a
cocktail glass. Garnish with a sage sprig and a lime wedge. Feel free
to add a squeeze of lime juice from the wedge for a tangier version.

21 GRAPE EXPECTATIONS

10 green grapes, plus extra for garnish
2 ounces fresh sour (see page 11)
1 ounce dry vermouth
1 ounce gin

Combine the grapes, fresh sour, vermouth, and gin in a blender and
blend for about 5 seconds. Add about 1 cup of ice and blend until
smooth. Pour into a cocktail glass. Garnish with green grapes.

22 GOODNESS GRAPENESS

15 green grapes, plus 2 for garnish
1 ounce citrus vodka (or grape vodka)
1 ounce brut champagne (i.e. Chandon Brut)
¾ ounce St-Germain elderflower liqueur
½ ounce simple syrup (see page 7)
½ ounce fresh lime juice

Combine the 15 grapes, vodka, champagne, elderflower liqueur, simple syrup, and lime juice in a blender and blend for about 5 seconds. Add about 1 cup of ice and blend until smooth. Pour into a champagne flute and garnish with 2 skewered green grapes.

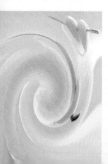

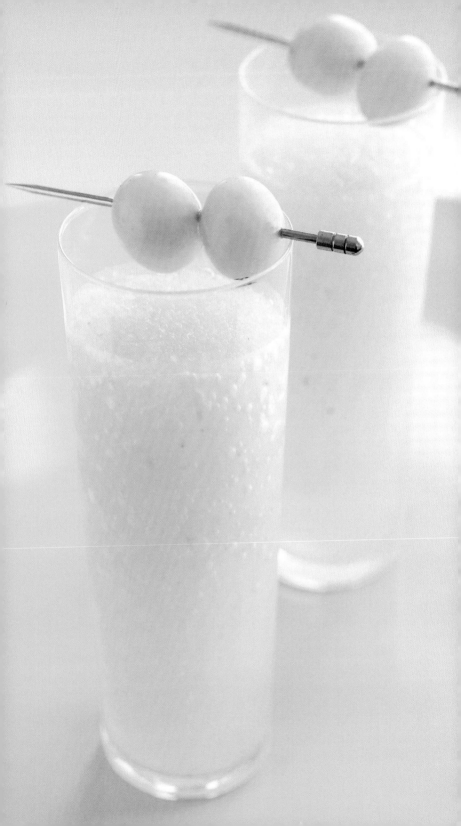

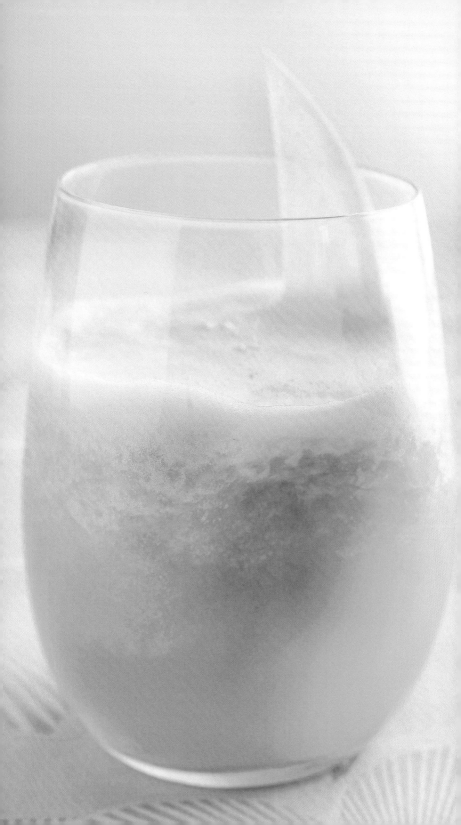

23 GREEN-EYED LADY

MAKES 1 TO 2 SERVINGS

1½ cups fresh honeydew melon chunks
4 ounces fresh sour (see page 11)
1 ounce absinthe (or pastis)
1 ounce Midori
1 or 2 small honeydew melon wedges, for garnish

Combine the melon, fresh sour, absinthe, and Midori in a blender
and blend for about 5 seconds. Add about 1 cup of ice and blend
until smooth. Pour into a cocktail glass. Garnish with a melon wedge.

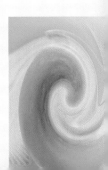

24 AU PEAR SIPPER

3 ounces pear nectar
1½ ounces Hendrick's gin
1 ounce hibiscus orange syrup (see page 8, or Monin also
    makes a Hibiscus syrup)
Dash of fresh lemon juice
Small lemon twist, for garnish

Combine the pear nectar, gin, syrup, and lemon juice in a blender
with 3 or 4 ice cubes. Blend until smooth. Pour into a cocktail glass.
Garnish with the lemon twist.

25 TAPIOCA THAI TEA

If you have not tried traditional Thai tea with the tapioca balls,
you're missing out. It's a bright orange sweetened tea mixed with
milk and extra-large tapioca balls that you suck out of a wide straw.
This is my cocktail version of this drink, served frozen.

⅓ cup tapioca pudding
2 ounces Thai tea
1 ounce dark rum, such as Bacardi 8
1 small scoop vanilla ice cream
Sage sprig, for garnish

Combine the tapioca pudding, tea, rum, and ice cream in a
blender and blend for about 5 seconds. Add about 1 cup of ice
and blend until smooth. Pour into a cocktail glass. Garnish with
the sprig of sage.

26 BANGKOK BANSHEE

½ banana, peeled
2 ounces Thai tea
1½ ounces dark rum, such as Bacardi 8
1 ounce simple syrup (see page 7)
1 ounce heavy whipping cream
Ground nutmeg, for garnish

Combine the banana, tea, rum, simple syrup, and cream in a blender and blend for about 5 seconds. Add about 1 cup of ice and blend until smooth. Pour into a cocktail glass and garnish with nutmeg.

27 SAKE TO ME

1½ ounces lychee juice or puree
1 ounce sake
1 ounce fresh sour (see page 11)
¾ ounce Zen green tea liqueur
Lychee nut and small stalk of lemongrass, for garnish

Combine the lychee juice, sake, fresh sour, and green tea liqueur in a blender and blend for about 5 seconds. Add about 1 cup of ice and blend until smooth. Pour into a cocktail glass. Garnish with the lychee nut and stalk of lemongrass.

28 YUZU-CUCUMBER FREEZE

1 ounce orange or citrus vodka
1 ounce sake
4 slices peeled cucumber
2 tablespoons yuzu marmalade
Cucumber spear and small orange wedge, for garnish

Combine the vodka, sake, cucumber slices, and marmalade in a blender and blend for about 5 seconds. Add about 1 cup of ice and blend until smooth. Pour into a glass. Garnish with the cucumber spear and orange wedge.

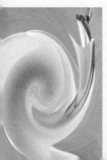

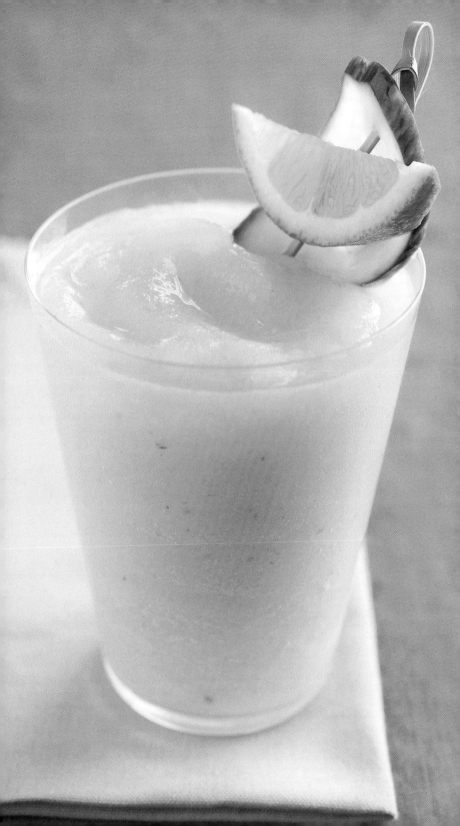

29 JASMINE PEACH BELLINI
MAKES 2 SERVINGS

3 ounces Prosecco
1½ ounces peach puree (or half a ripe peach, blanched, peeled,
    and cut into chunks)
1½ ounces jasmine tea syrup (see page 8)
1 ounce fresh lemon juice
2 lemon twists, for garnish

Combine the Prosecco, peach puree, tea syrup, and lemon juice in
a blender with 5 or 6 ice cubes. Blend until smooth. Pour into two
champagne flutes and garnish each with a lemon twist.

30 BLOOD PEACH BELLINI
MAKES 2 SERVINGS

2 ounces peach puree (or 1 ripe peach, blanched, peeled,
    and cut into chunks)
2 ounces Prosecco
1½ ounces blood orange juice
½ ounce peach liqueur
2 lemon twists, for garnish

Combine the peach puree, Prosecco, blood orange juice, and peach
liqueur in a blender with 5 or 6 ice cubes. Blend until smooth. Pour
into two champagne flutes and garnish each with a lemon twist.

31 FROZEN RUM PUNCH

1½ ounces dark rum
1 ounce orange juice
1 ounce pineapple juice
1 ounce cranberry juice
1 ounce coconut cream (such as Coco Lopez)
Maraschino cherry and orange wedge, for garnish

Combine the rum, orange juice, pineapple juice, cranberry juice, and coconut cream in a blender and blend for about 5 seconds. Add about 1 cup of ice and blend until smooth. Pour into a tall cocktail glass. Garnish with the cherry and orange wedge.

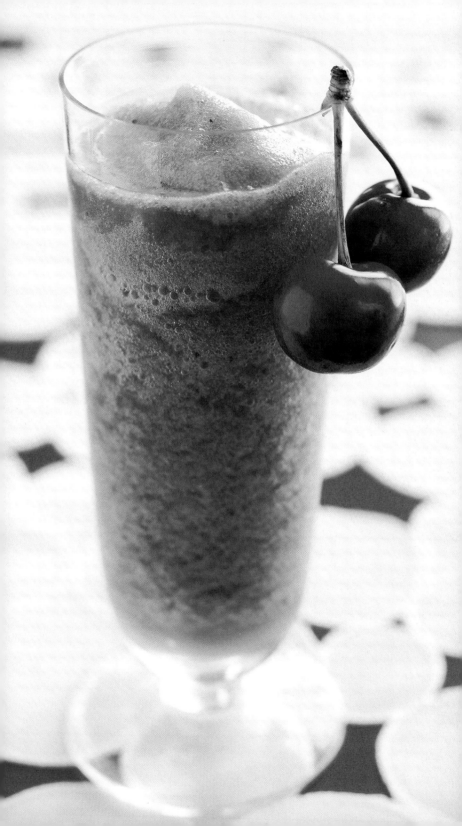

32 CHERRY SLING

2 ounces pineapple juice
1½ tablespoons black cherry preserves
1 ounce fresh sour (see page 11)
1 ounce gin
½ ounce Cherry Heering
¼ ounce Benedictine (or cognac)
Maraschino cherry and orange wedge, for garnish

Combine the pineapple juice, preserves, fresh sour, gin, Cherry Heering, and Benedictine in a blender and blend for about 5 seconds. Add about 1 cup of ice and blend until smooth. Pour into a Hurricane glass or other large glass and garnish with the cherry and orange wedge.

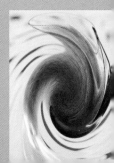

33 GRANDMA'S FROZEN APRICOT

2 ounces apricot nectar (such as Kern's)
2 ounces orange juice
1 ounce Grand Marnier
2 tablespoons apricot preserves
Splash of fresh lemon juice
Freshly grated orange zest and mint sprig, for garnish

Combine the apricot nectar, orange juice, Grand Marnier, apricot preserves, and lemon juice in a blender and blend for about 5 seconds. Add about 1 cup of ice and blend until smooth. Pour into a cocktail glass and garnish with the orange zest and mint sprig.

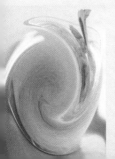

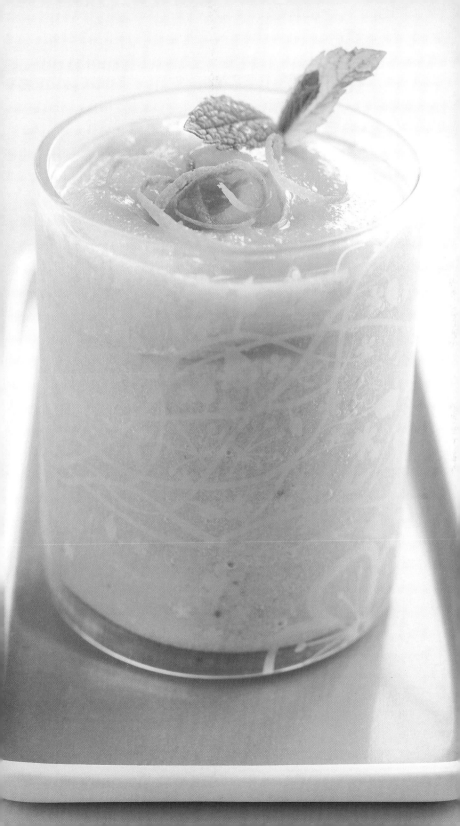

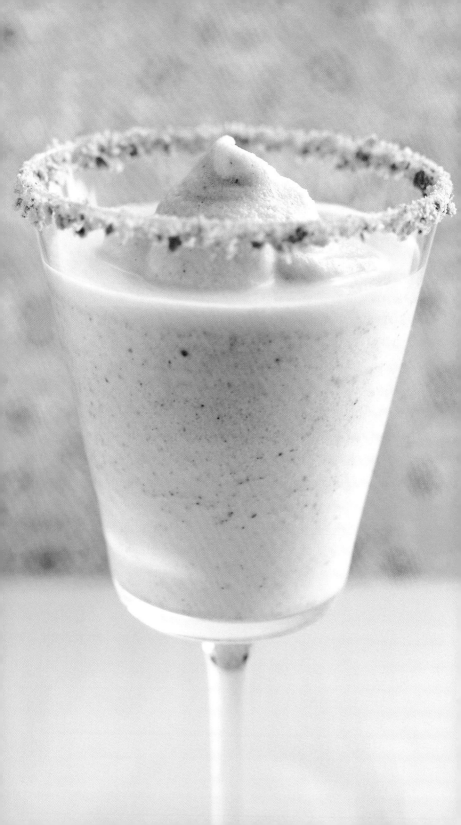

34 GRAHAM SLAM

Simple syrup (see page 7; optional)
Graham cracker crumbs, for garnishing rim (optional)
1 large scoop vanilla ice cream
2 graham cracker squares (preferably cinnamon-coated)
1½ ounces bourbon
Dash of cinnamon (optional)
Milk, if needed

If desired, wet the rim of a cocktail glass with simple syrup and dip it into a plate of graham cracker crumbs. Set aside.

Combine the ice cream, graham cracker squares, bourbon, and cinnamon, if desired, in a blender and blend for about 5 seconds. Add about 1 cup of ice and blend until smooth. (Add a little milk if the ice cream is too hard.) Pour into the cocktail glass.

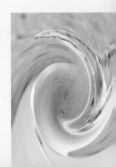

35 FROZEN BLACK WHIP

Inspired by the Black Flip cocktail I had at PDT ("Please don't tell") by Jim Meehan in NYC. Sooooooo goooood.

1 large scoop vanilla ice cream
2 ounces Guinness
1 ounce Cruzan Black Strap rum
Ground nutmeg, for garnish

Combine the ice cream, Guinness, and rum in a blender and blend for about 5 seconds. Add about a half cup of ice and blend until smooth. Pour into a small cocktail glass and top with nutmeg.

36 MELLOW YELLOW

½ banana, peeled
2 ounces limoncello
2 ounces orange juice
1 ounce milk

Combine the banana, limoncello, orange juice, and milk in a blender and blend for about 5 seconds. Add about 1 cup of ice and blend until smooth. Pour into a cocktail glass.

37 BACHATA

From master mixologist Bridget Albert.

4 fresh watermelon cubes
1½ ounces Malibu passion fruit rum
1 ounce pink grapefruit juice
Juice of 1 lime

In a blender, blend 2 to 3 cups of ice cubes to make shaved ice. Add the shaved ice to a glass or snow cone cup. In a cocktail shaker, muddle (mash) the watermelon cubes. Add the rum, grapefruit juice, and lime juice, add ice cubes, and shake. Pour over the shaved ice.

38 PINK FLAMINGO ICE

4 ounces ruby red grapefruit juice
1½ ounces X-Rated liqueur (a mango, passion fruit, and blood orange liqueur)
½ ounce Aperol (an Italian bitters similar to Campari, but much milder)
½ ounce simple syrup (see page 7)
Small grapefruit wedge, for garnish

Combine the grapefruit juice, X-Rated liqueur, Aperol, and simple syrup in a blender with 5 or 6 ice cubes. Blend until smooth. Pour into a cocktail glass and garnish with the grapefruit wedge.

39 PURPLE HAZE

1 cup seasonal berries of your choice
2 ounces Chambord
2 ounces white cranberry juice
Light purple or white orchid, for garnish

Combine the berries, Chambord, and cranberry juice in a blender and blend for about 5 seconds. Add about 1 cup of ice and blend until smooth. Pour into a cocktail glass. Garnish with the orchid.

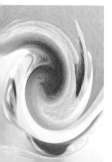

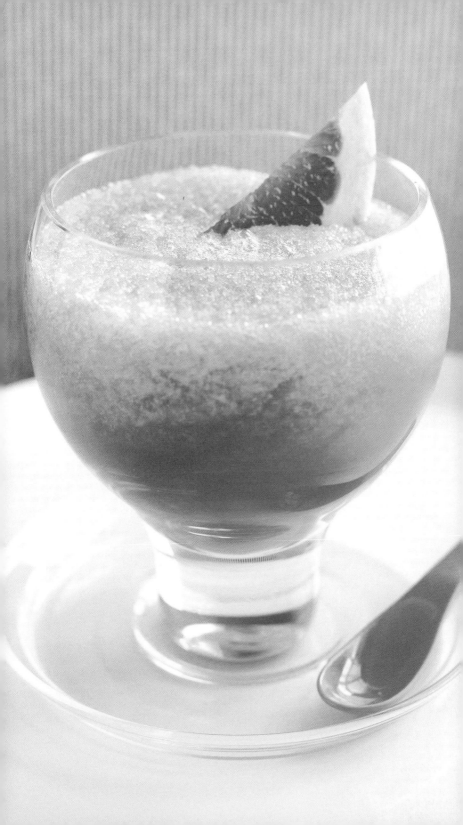

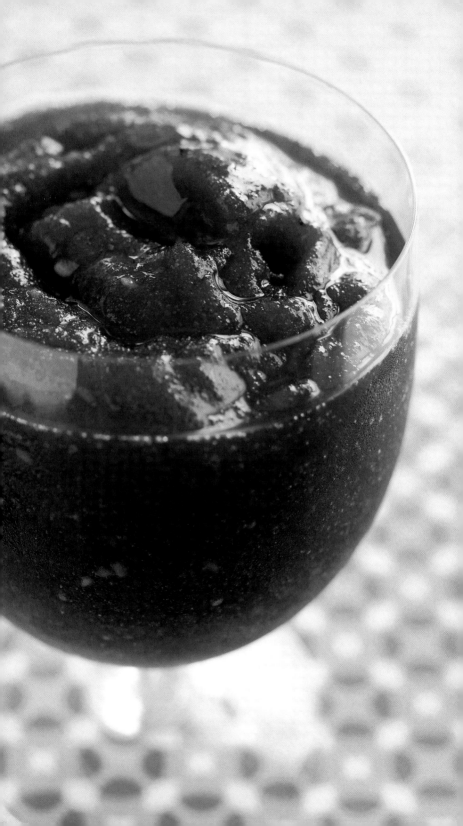

40 BLACKBERRY BRAMBLICIOUS

5 blackberries
1½ ounces gin
1 ounce simple syrup (see page 7)
¾ ounce fresh lime juice
½ ounce crème de cassis

Combine the blackberries, gin, simple syrup, lime juice, and crème de cassis in a blender and blend for about 5 seconds. Add about 1 cup of ice and blend until smooth. Pour into a cocktail glass.

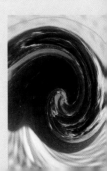

41 PIMM'S FREEZE

4 cucumber slices
2 strawberries
4 ounces ginger ale
1½ ounces Pimm's No. 1
Cucumber spear, strawberry, and mint sprig, for garnish

Combine the cucumber slices, strawberries, ginger ale, and Pimm's in a blender and blend for about 5 seconds. Add about 1 cup of ice and blend until smooth. Pour into a cocktail glass. Garnish with the cucumber spear, strawberry, and mint sprig.

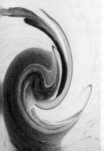

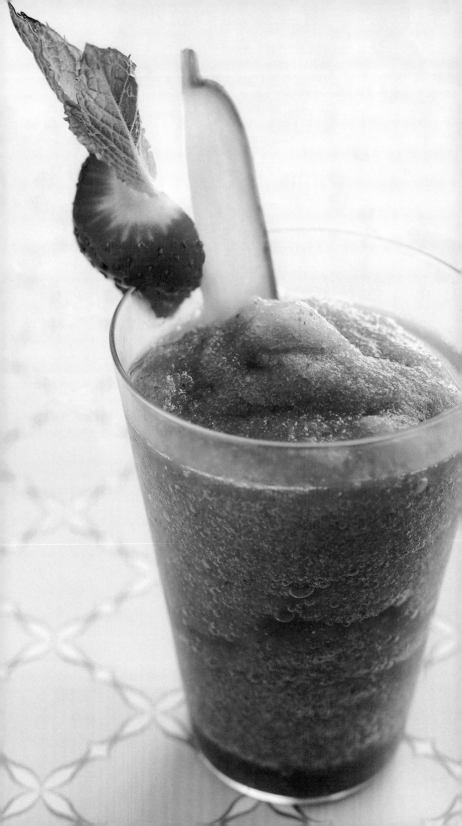

42 BEET AROUND THE BUSH

A variation on master mixologist Bridget Albert's Spiced Beet Cocktail, from her book *Market Fresh Mixology* (Surrey Books, 2008).

> 1 beet, peeled and sliced
> Juice of 3 limes
> 2 teaspoons brown sugar
> Pinch of ground ginger
> 1½ ounces silver tequila
> 1 ounce simple syrup (see page 7)
> 1 ounce fresh lemon juice
> ½ ounce mescal
> Piece of beet leaf, for garnish (cut it in halves or quarters
>   to fit in the glass, if needed.)

In a sauté pan, combine the beet, lime juice, brown sugar, and ginger. Cover and simmer over medium heat, stirring occasionally, until the beets are tender, about 10 minutes. Remove the beets and discard (or keep for eating later) and let the liquid cool. Pour the liquid into a blender and add the tequila, simple syrup, lemon juice, and mescal. Blend for about 5 seconds then add about 1 cup of ice and blend until smooth. Pour into a cocktail glass and garnish with the beet leaf.

43 BLUEBERRY BLITZ

I'm a big fan of Tyler Florence—in fact, my husband refers to
his *Tyler's Ultimate* book (Clarkson Potter, 2006) as our "Go-To
Cookbook" for great recipes. This recipe is inspired by one of his
creations, a blueberry blintz.

  10 blueberries, plus 4 for garnish
  1 tablespoon mascarpone cheese
  1 ounce simple syrup (see page 7)
  1 ounce Chambord
  Dash of vanilla extract (⅛ teaspoon)

Combine the 10 blueberries, mascarpone, simple syrup, Chambord,
and vanilla extract in a blender and blend for about 5 seconds. Add
about a half cup of ice and blend until smooth. Pour into a cocktail
glass and garnish with 4 skewered blueberries.

44 LINGONBERRIES FALLING DOWN

  2 tablespoons lingonberry preserves
  1 ounce orange vodka
  1 ounce orange juice
  ½ ounce fresh sour (see page 11)
  Large piece of orange peel, for garnish

Combine the preserves, vodka, orange juice, and fresh sour in a
blender for about 5 seconds. Add about a half cup of ice and blend
until smooth. Pour into a cocktail glass. Garnish with the orange peel.

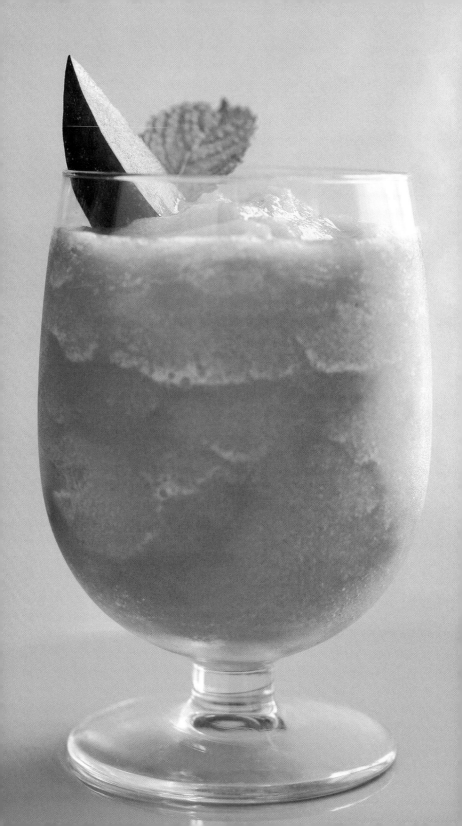

45 PLUM DIGGITY

Inspired by Jamie Oliver's Plums & Sloe Gin recipe.

2 plums (blanched, peeled, and cut into chunks)
4 ounces orange juice (best, if freshly squeezed)
1½ ounces sloe gin
Plum slice and mint sprig, for garnish

Combine the plums, orange juice, and gin in a blender and blend for about 5 seconds. Add about a half cup of ice and blend until smooth. Pour into a cocktail glass and garnish with the plum slice and mint sprig.

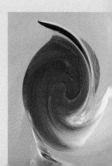

46 PASSION FRUIT MOUSSE

Recipe by Todd Appel, a mixologist from Chicago, Illinois.

    2 ounces cachaça or light rum
    1½ ounces sweetened condensed milk
    Pulp of 1 medium fresh passion fruit (seeds reserved for garnish,
      if desired), or 1 ounce passion fruit puree or syrup

Combine the cachaça, milk, and passion fruit pulp in a blender
with 1 cup of ice. Blend until smooth. You can adjust the amount
of condensed milk to your taste, depending on the size and tartness
of the passion fruit. Pour into a tall Collins glass with a long straw
and enjoy! Seeds of passion fruit are fine to eat and add some visual
appeal to the cocktail.

47 FROZEN CHERRY COKE

    4 ounces Coke
    1½ ounces SKYY Cherry vodka
    1 ounce cherry syrup (such as Monin)
    Fresh or maraschino cherry, for garnish

Combine the Coke, vodka, and cherry syrup in a blender with 5 to
7 ice cubes. Blend until smooth. Pour into a tall glass and garnish
with the cherry. Serve with a straw.

48 TRUE BLUE

2 ounces pineapple juice
2 ounces orange juice
1 ounce blue curaçao
1 ounce rum
Orange quarter-wheel, for garnish

Combine the pineapple juice, orange juice, curaçao, and rum in a blender with 1 cup of ice. Blend until smooth. Pour into a cocktail glass and garnish with the orange quarter-wheel.

49 TREE HUGGER

MAKES 2 SMALL SERVINGS OR 1 LARGE SERVING

I created this for my brother, Brian, a true tree-hugger. This cocktail is made with TRU vanilla vodka (a carbon-negative vodka)—the company actually plants a tree for every bottle sold!

½ banana, peeled
¼ cup organic granola, plus extra for garnish
1 large scoop vanilla ice cream (organic if possible)
1½ ounces TRU vanilla vodka
Soy milk (optional)
Chocolate chips, for garnish

Combine the banana, granola, ice cream, and vodka in a blender and blend for about 5 seconds. Add about a half cup of ice and blend until smooth, adding soy milk if the ice cream is too hard. Pour into two small juice glasses or one larger glass. Sprinkle the top with granola and chocolate chips for garnish.

50 GRILLED PEACH MELBA

1 peach, peeled, cut in half, pitted, and grilled
1½ ounces sweetened condensed milk
1 ounce milk
1 ounce cognac (or brandy)
Dash of cinnamon, for garnish

Combine the grilled peach, condensed milk, regular milk, and cognac in a blender and blend for about 5 seconds. Add about 1 cup of ice and blend until smooth. Pour into a cocktail glass and garnish with the cinnamon.

51 FIG 'N' HONEY

3 to 4 ounces orange juice
1 tablespoon fig marmalade
1 ounce cognac
½ teaspoon clover honey
½ fig, for garnish (fresh or dried, whichever is available)

Combine the orange juice, marmalade, cognac, and honey in a blender and blend for about 5 seconds. Add about 1 cup of ice and blend until smooth. Pour into a cocktail glass and garnish with the fig half.

52 CAPETA PEQUENO NOVO (NEW LITTLE DEMON)

Created by one of my mixologist friends in Chicago, Kyle McHugh of TheBoozehound.com. He created this drink as a way to do something different with cachaça and to really capture the Brazilian lifestyle. (The guarana powder may be left out if you are unable to find it.)

2 ounces skim milk
1½ ounces cinnamon-infused Leblon cachaça
1 ounce sweetened condensed milk
1 ounce coconut milk
1 tablespoon clover honey
1 teaspoon unsalted blanched peanuts
1 teaspoon guarana powder
1 teaspoon 100 percent cocoa powder (or chocolate shavings)

Combine the skim milk, cachaça, condensed milk, coconut milk, honey, peanuts, guarana powder, and cocoa powder in a blender with a few ice cubes. Blend on high for 30 seconds. Pour into a cocktail glass.

53 PERUVIAN PINEAPPLE

Created by mixologist Natalie Bovis-Nelson, The Liquid Muse.

¼ cup roasted fresh pineapple chunks
2 ounces Peruvian pisco
1 ounce honey water (see page 7)
¾ ounce heavy whipping cream
½ ounce fresh lime juice
¼ teaspoon nutmeg, plus a tiny pinch for garnish
Pineapple wedge, for garnish

Combine the pineapple, pisco, honey water, cream, lime juice, and nutmeg in a blender. Blend for 15 seconds, then add a quarter cup of crushed ice. Blend until smooth. Pour into a wine goblet or large martini glass. Garnish with a sprinkle of nutmeg and the pineapple wedge.

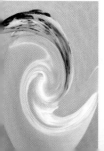

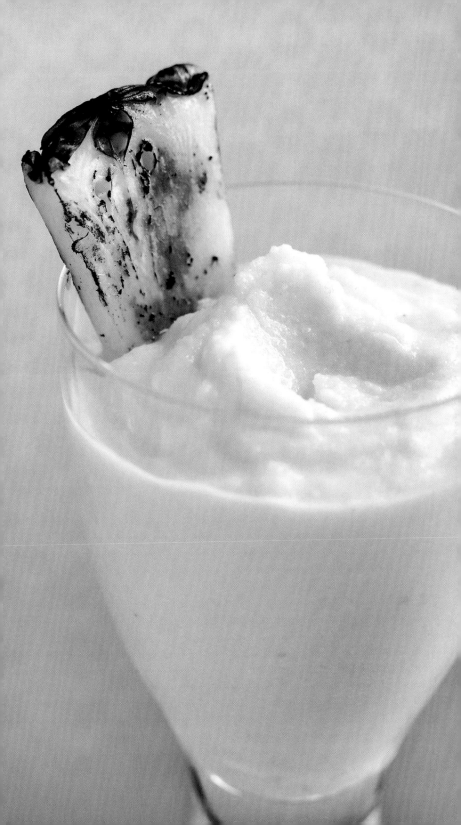

54 CARAMELIZED PEAR MACERATE

1 Bosc pear
1 ounce simple syrup (see page 7)
Dash of ground nutmeg, plus extra for garnish
Dash of ground cinnamon
2 ounces cognac
⅛ teaspoon vanilla extract
2 ounces heavy whipping cream

Peel the pear, core it, and cut into thin slices (save 2 of the slices for the garnish). In a sauté pan over medium heat, sauté the pear slices with the simple syrup, nutmeg, and cinnamon until the pear slices become soft. (You may need to add additional simple syrup to prevent the pear slices from sticking to the pan.) Add the cognac and vanilla and scrape everything into a blender. Add the cream and blend for about 5 seconds. Add about a half cup of ice and blend until smooth. Pour into a small cocktail glass. Garnish with the pear slices and a dash of nutmeg.

55 SASSY SUZETTE

Inspired by the classic crêpes suzette.

1 scoop vanilla ice cream
1 ounce maple syrup
1 ounce sweetened condensed milk
1 ounce bourbon
½ ounce Grand Marnier

Combine the ice cream, maple syrup, milk, and bourbon in a blender and blend for about 5 seconds. Add about a half cup of ice and blend smooth. (If desired, add more bourbon.) Pour into a cocktail glass and top with the Grand Marnier.

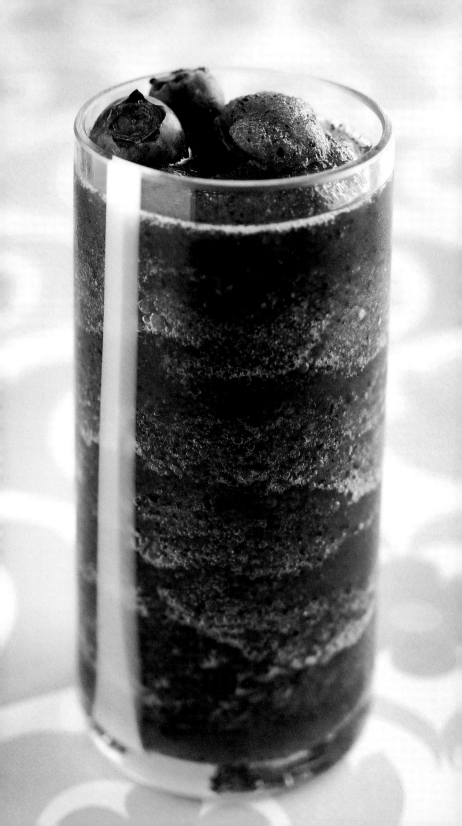

56 TYPHOON

10 blueberries
2 ounces pineapple juice
2 ounces fresh sour (see page 11)
1½ ounces SKYY passion fruit vodka
1 ounce blue curaçao

Combine the blueberries, pineapple juice, fresh sour, vodka, and curaçao in a blender and blend for about 5 seconds. Add about a half cup of ice and blend until smooth. Pour into a tall cocktail glass.

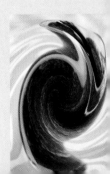

57 PANDA FREEZE

1 scoop vanilla ice cream
2 ounces Baileys mint chocolate liqueur
½ ounce white crème de menthe (or peppermint schnapps)
¼ cup chocolate chips

Combine the ice cream, Baileys, and crème de menthe in a blender and blend for about 5 seconds. Add about a half cup of ice and blend until smooth. (If the ice cream is too soft, add a few more ice cubes to make it thicker.) Add the chocolate chips and blend for 2 seconds (just enough to fold them into the mix). Pour into a tall glass.

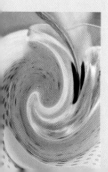

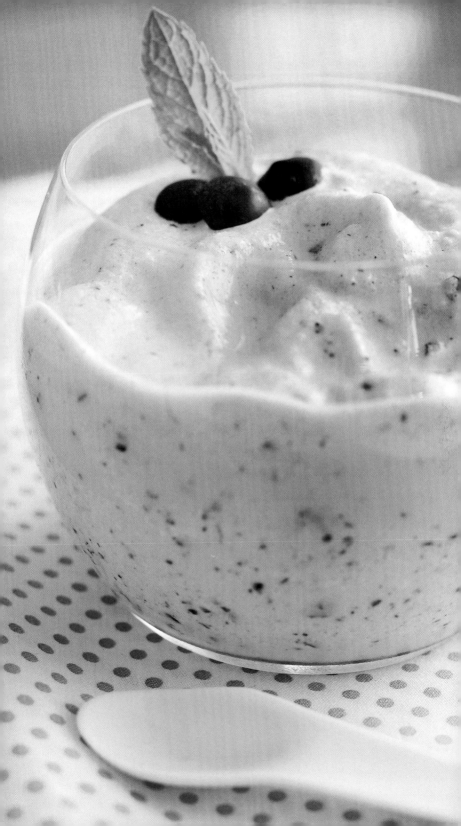

58 TIDDLIWINK

15 blueberries
4 ounces orange juice
1½ ounces mango rum
½ cups fresh mango chunks

Combine the blueberries, orange juice, rum, and mango chunks in a blender and blend on high for 10 seconds. Add 5 or 6 ice cubes and blend until smooth. Pour into a cocktail glass.

59 PEACHES 'N' CREAM

1 ripe peach (blanched, peeled, and cut into chunks)
1 scoop vanilla ice cream
1 ounce Navan vanilla liqueur
½ ounce peach liqueur

Combine the peach chunks, ice cream, vanilla liqueur, and peach liqueur in a blender and blend on high for 10 seconds. Add 5 or 6 ice cubes and blend until smooth. Pour into a cocktail glass.

60 BANANAS FOSTER FRAPPE

MAKES 8 SERVINGS

From master mixologist Jonathan Pogash, The Cocktail Guru, NYC.

3 bananas, peeled
1/3 cup raw sugar (turbinado sugar)
Juice of 1/2 lemon
1/2 ounce Grand Marnier
1/4 teaspoon ground cinnamon
3 cups low-fat vanilla ice cream (slightly softened)
3/4 cup Mount Gay Eclipse rum
3/4 cup low-fat or fat-free half-and-half
1/2 teaspoon banana extract
Sliced strawberries, for garnish

Preheat the oven to 300°F. Spray a baking dish with nonstick cooking spray. Slice the bananas lengthwise and then into 1-inch chunks. Add the bananas to a mixing bowl along with the sugar, lemon juice, Grand Marnier, and cinnamon. Toss gently. Place the banana mixture into the baking dish and cook until softened, about 10 minutes. Allow to cool thoroughly.

Add the cooled banana mixture and accumulated syrup to a blender along with the ice cream, rum, half-and-half, and banana extract. Blend until smooth. Pour into eight chilled wine goblets. Garnish with sliced strawberries.

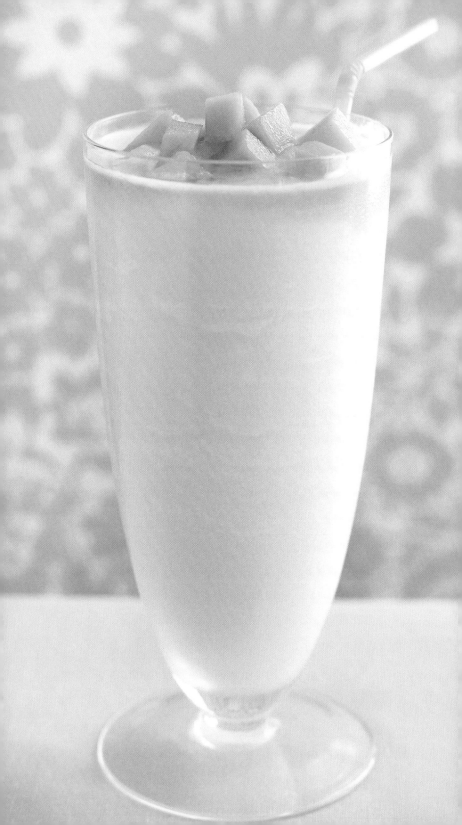

61 KIM'S ULTIMATE PIÑA COLADA

2 ounces coconut cream (such as Coco Lopez)
2 ounces pineapple juice
1½ ounces coconut rum
Splash of heavy whipping cream
¼ cup chopped fresh mango
½ ounce spiced rum or Navan vanilla liqueur

Combine the coconut cream, pineapple juice, rum, and cream in a blender and blend on high for 10 seconds. Add 5 to 7 ice cubes and blend until smooth. Pour into a tall Hurricane glass or other large glass. Top with the chopped mango and float the spiced rum on top.

62 THAI COLADA

Follow the recipe above, but omit the spiced rum float and chopped mango. Blend in ½ teaspoon ground cardamom and top with ground nutmeg.

63 COCOA COLADA

This is the same recipe as the Thai Colada, but substitute 1 tablespoon unsweetened cocoa powder for the cardamom. Top with shaved chocolate as an optional garnish.

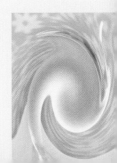

64 FROZEN PEACH JULEP

2 ounces bourbon
1½ ounces white peach syrup (such as Monin)
2 or 3 mint leaves
½ cup fresh peaches, peeled and chopped (optional)
Dash of fresh lemon juice
Mint sprig, for garnish

Combine the bourbon, white peach syrup, mint leaves, and peaches, if desired, and lemon juice in a blender and blend for about 5 seconds. Add about 1 cup of ice and blend with 5 to 7 ice cubes. Blend until smooth. Pour into a rocks glass and garnish with the mint sprig.

65 FROZEN MOJITO

2 ounces rum
1½ ounces fresh lime juice
1½ ounces simple syrup (see page 7)
3 or 4 mint leaves
Mint sprig, for garnish

Combine the rum, lime juice, simple syrup, and mint leaves in a blender with 5 to 7 ice cubes. Blend until smooth. Pour into a cocktail glass and garnish with the mint sprig.

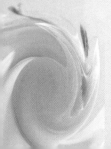

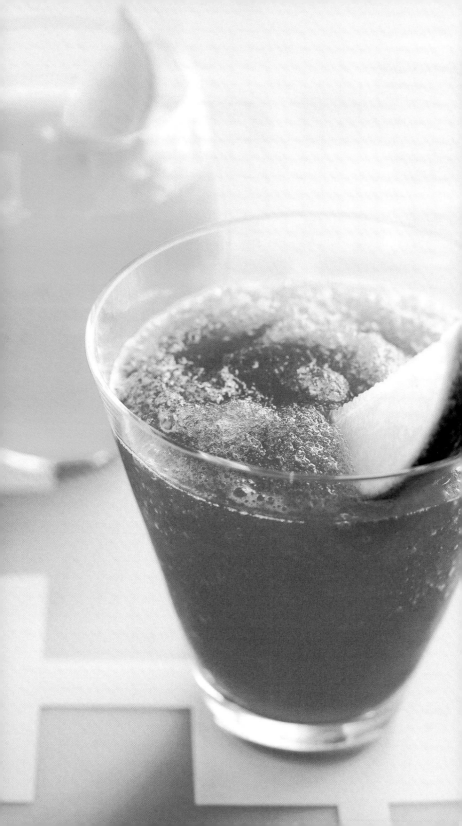

66 FROZEN COSMOPOLITAN

2 ounces cranberry juice
1½ ounces orange or citrus vodka
¾ ounce triple sec
½ ounce fresh lime juice
Lime wedge, for garnish

Combine the cranberry juice, vodka, triple sec, and lime juice in a blender with 4 or 5 ice cubes. Blend until smooth. Pour into a martini glass and garnish with the lime wedge.

67 FROZEN BLUE COSMOPOLITAN

Use the same recipe as above, but substitute blue curaçao for the triple sec and white cranberry juice for the red.

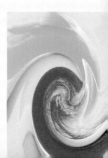

68 FROZEN SANGRIA
MAKES 3 SERVINGS

From my book 101 *Sangrias and Pitcher Drinks*.

2 cups red wine
1 cup simple syrup (see page 7)
1 cup frozen fruit chunks (such as peaches, berries, apples, grapes, pineapple, etc.)
4 ounces Cointreau
4 ounces Ballatore Gran Spumante
3 orange wheels, for garnish

Combine the wine, simple syrup, fruit, Cointreau, and spumante in a blender with 5 to 7 ice cubes. Blend until smooth. Pour into three wine goblets and garnish each with an orange wheel.

69 SPECKLEBERRY SANGRIA
MAKES 4 SERVINGS

2 cups white zinfandel
4 ounces fresh lime juice
4 ounces orange juice
4 ounces simple syrup (see page 7)
4 ounces orange curaçao
¼ cup chopped fresh pineapple
5 blueberries
3 raspberries
4 lime wheels, for garnish

Combine the zinfandel, lime juice, orange juice, simple syrup, curaçao, pineapple, blueberries, and raspberries in a blender and blend for about 5 seconds. Add about 1 cup of ice and blend until smooth. Pour into four wine goblets and garnish each with a lime wheel.

70 TROPICAL BLUSH SANGRIA

3 ounces sauvignon blanc
1 ounce X-Rated liqueur
1 ounce passion fruit syrup
1 ounce pineapple juice
1 ounce 7-Up
½ ounce SKYY Infusions pineapple vodka
Pineapple wedge, for garnish

Combine the sauvignon blanc, X-Rated liqueur, passion fruit syrup, pineapple juice, 7-Up, and vodka in a blender for about 5 seconds. Add about 1 cup of ice and blend until smooth. Pour into a wine goblet. Garnish with the pineapple wedge.

71 EVERYDAY FRUIT SANGRIA

Inspired by Giada De Laurentiis's "Everyday Fruit" chapter in her book, *Everyday Italian* (Clarkson Potter, 2005).

1 cup sweet riesling
½ cup chopped fresh cantaloupe, plus extra for garnish
2 strawberries, stems removed, plus extra for garnish
10 to 15 red and white grapes, plus extra for garnish
3 mint leaves
Splash of Sprite

Combine the riesling, cantaloupe, strawberries, grapes, mint leaves, and Sprite in a blender and blend for about 5 seconds. Add about 1 cup of ice and blend until smooth. Pour into a wine goblet. Garnish with skewered fruit.

72 MIDNIGHT SANGRIA

MAKES 2 SERVINGS

2 cups red zinfandel
1 cup orange juice
2 ounces 7-Up
5 blackberries, plus extra for garnish
10 to 15 blueberries, plus extra for garnish
2 ounces blueberry syrup (such as Monin)

Combine the zinfandel, orange juice, 7-Up, blackberries, blueberries, and blueberry syrup in a blender and blend for about 5 seconds. Add about 1 cup of ice and blend until smooth. Pour into two wine goblets. Garnish with skewered blackberries and blueberries.

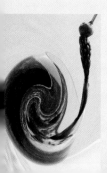

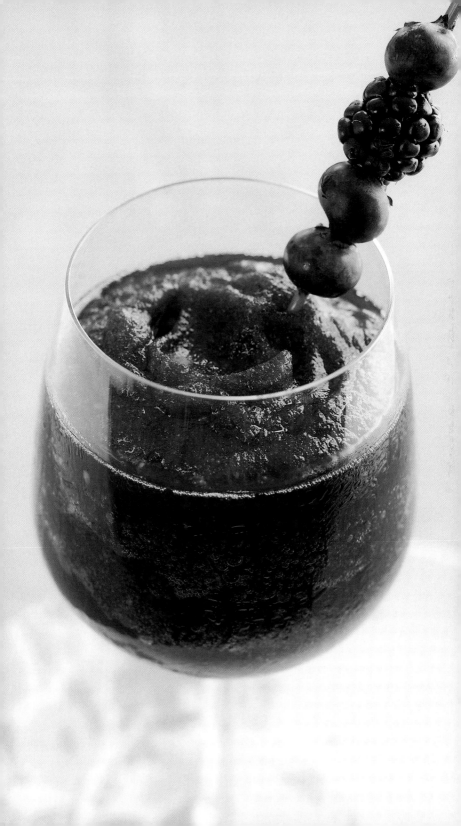

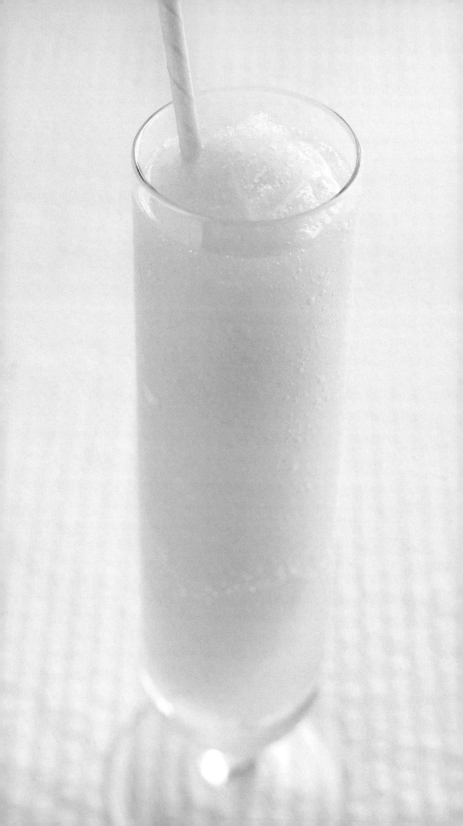

73 FROZEN BELLINI

½ cup peeled and chopped peaches
3 ounces sweet sparkling wine
1 ounce peach liqueur
½ ounce simple syrup (see page 7)

Combine the peaches, sparkling wine, peach liqueur, and simple syrup in a blender and blend for about 5 seconds. Add about 1 cup of ice and blend until smooth. Pour into a cocktail glass or champagne flute.

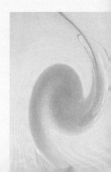

74 FROZEN BERRY BELLINI

½ cup mixed berries (fresh or frozen)
2 to 3 ounces sparkling wine (sweet, preferred)
1 ounce simple syrup (see page 7)
1 ounce pineapple juice

Combine the berries, sparkling wine, simple syrup, and pineapple juice in a blender and blend for about 5 seconds. Add about 1 cup of ice and blend until smooth. Pour into a cocktail glass or champagne flute.

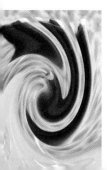

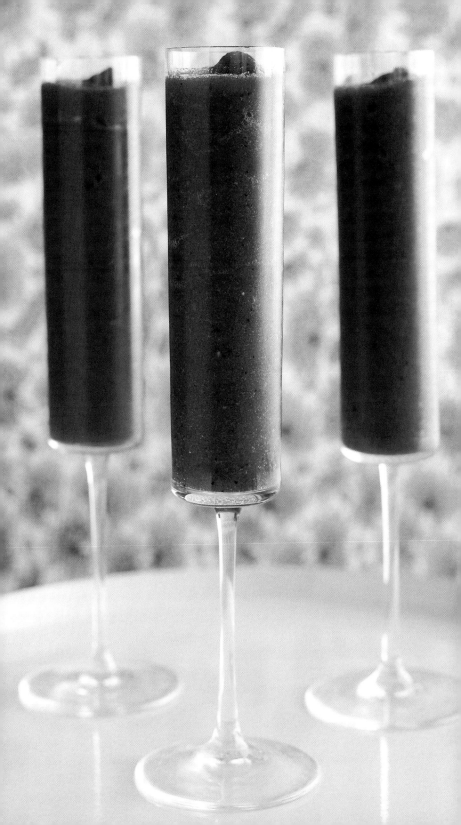

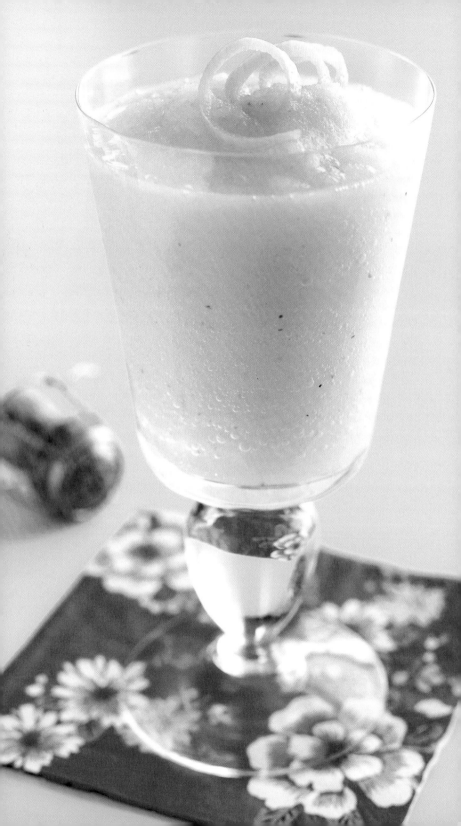

75 SHANGHAI BLOSSOM BELLINI

2 to 3 ounces sweet sparkling wine
2 ounces lychee puree (or juice)
½ ounce St-Germain elderflower liqueur
½ ounce citrus vodka
Splash of fresh lemon juice
Lemon twist, for garnish

Combine the sparkling wine, lychee puree, elderflower liqueur, vodka, and lemon juice in a blender and blend for about 5 seconds. Add about 1 cup of ice and blend until smooth. Pour into a champagne flute and garnish with the lemon twist.

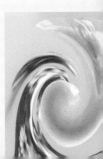

76 CRANTOPIA CRUSH

3 ounces orange juice
1½ ounces orange vodka
1 ounce cranberry juice
¾ ounce Cointreau
2 tablespoons cranberry sauce (best if homemade)
3 whole cranberries and mint sprig, for garnish

Combine the orange juice, vodka, cranberry juice, Cointreau, and cranberry sauce in a blender and blend for about 5 seconds. Add about 1 cup of ice and blend until smooth. Pour into a cocktail glass. Garnish with the cranberries and mint sprig.

77 SHIVERING YELLOW BULL

For all you die-hard "vodka & Red Bull" fans, this is a good fresh frozen version.

2 ounces Red Bull
2 ounces fresh sour (see page 11)
1½ ounces citrus or grapefruit vodka
1 ounce passion fruit puree
Orange wedge, for garnish

Combine the Red Bull, fresh sour, vodka, and passion fruit puree in a blender and blend for about 5 seconds. Add about 1 cup of ice and blend until smooth. Pour into a cocktail glass and garnish with the orange wedge.

78 DETOX DAZE

A detoxifying elixir to help you ramp up again after a long night.

1 banana, peeled
2 kiwis, peeled
4 ounces soy milk
2 tablespoons protein powder
1 dandelion root, dried (can be purchased in health or herbal stores)
1 dropper-full ginseng
1 dropper-full milk thistle

Combine the banana, kiwis, soy milk, protein powder, dandelion root, ginseng, and milk thistle in a blender and blend for about 5 seconds. Add about 1 cup of ice and blend until smooth. Pour into a tall glass.

79 FLIP FLOP (AKA BAR-TENDER'S BREAKFAST SHOT)

Many bartenders do digestif shots behind the bar as a way to calm upset stomachs and clear the head. This is a morning breakfast drink, with a good dose of vitamin C, protein, and caffeine, and it's pretty darned good.

3 ounces digestif of choice (such as Fernet-Branca, Averna, etc.)
1 whole egg
Juice of 1 orange
Shot of coffee (or espresso)

Combine the digestif, egg, orange juice, and coffee in a blender and blend for about 5 seconds. Add a few cubes of ice and blend until smooth. Pour into a juice glass.

80 ANTIOX POM CRUSH

Chock-full of antioxidants.

10 blueberries
4 black cherries
2 ounces acai juice
1½ ounces SKYY cherry vodka
1 ounce pomegranate juice

Combine the blueberries, cherries, acai juice, vodka, and pome-granate juice in a blender and blend for about 5 seconds. Add about 1 cup of ice and blend until smooth. Pour into a cocktail glass.

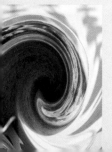

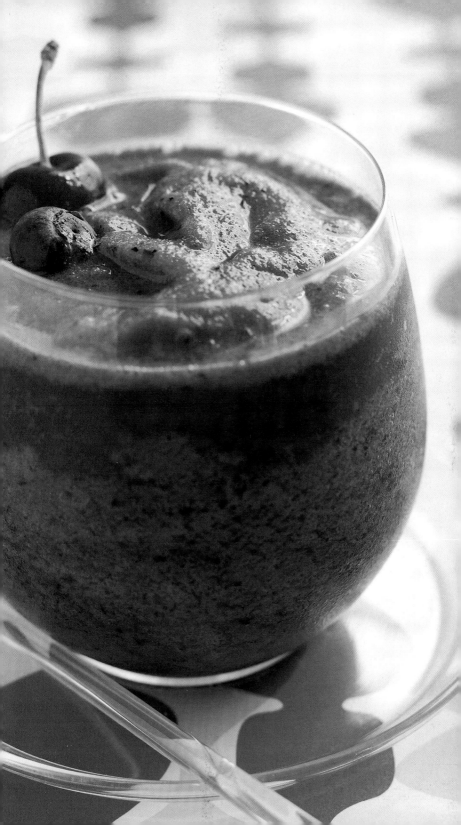

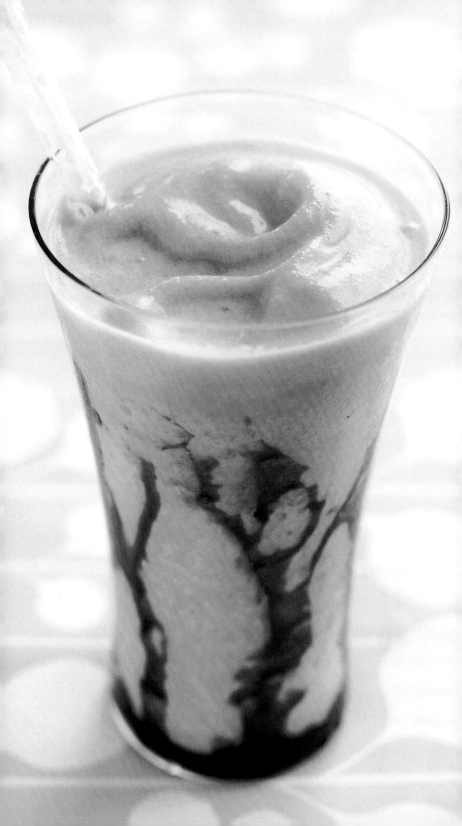

81 CHOCOLATE MONKEY

Chocolate syrup
½ banana, peeled
1 large scoop vanilla ice cream
1½ ounces Godiva chocolate liqueur
1 ounce crème de banana

Swirl the chocolate syrup down the sides of a tall glass and set aside.
Combine the banana, ice cream, chocolate liqueur, crème de banana, and a good squeeze of chocolate syrup in a blender and blend
for about 5 seconds. Add about 1 cup of ice and blend until smooth.
Pour into the swirled glass. Serve with a straw.

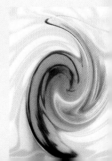

82 MUDSPLASH

I developed this cocktail with SKYY Spirits in conjunction with the television series *Wipeout*, a show filled with very messy, muddy stunts.

Chocolate syrup
3 gingersnap cookies
1 large scoop vanilla ice cream
1 ounce Cabo Wabo Tequila Blanco
1 ounce light cream
Whipped cream and a gingerbread man cookie, for garnish

Swirl the chocolate syrup down the sides of a tall glass and set aside. Combine the cookies, ice cream, tequila, and light cream in a blender and blend for about 5 seconds. Add about a half cup of ice and blend until smooth. Pour into the swirled glass. Top with whipped cream. Place the gingerbread man in the whipped cream (as if he were drowning in the drink).

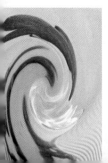

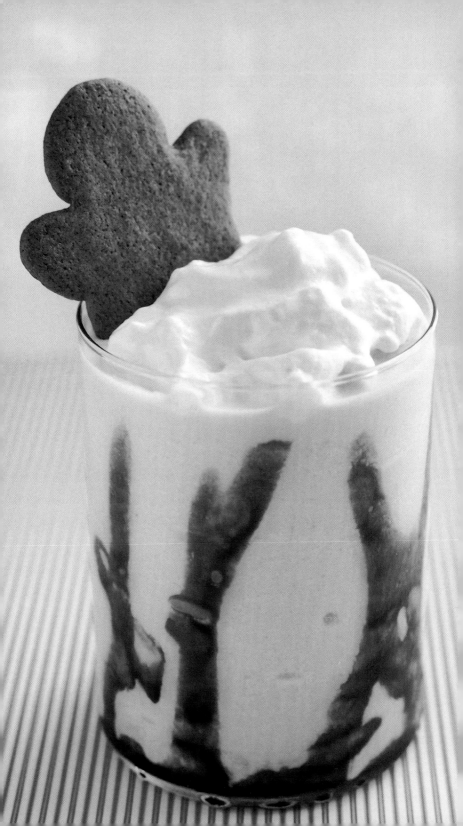

83 FROZEN WHITE RUSSIAN

This is actually more like a Frozen Sombrero because it's layered, but it's a great dessert drink.

1 soft brownie
1 large scoop vanilla ice cream
1 ounce Baileys Irish Cream
1 ounce vanilla vodka

Mash the brownie in the bottom of a rocks glass. Combine the ice cream, Baileys, and vodka in a blender and blend for about 5 seconds. Add a few cubes of ice and blend until smooth. Pour on top of the mashed brownie and serve with a spoon.

84 CHOCOLATE NARCISSA

For chocoholics united, especially Diane who eats Oreos for breakfast.

1 large scoop chocolate ice cream
4 chocolate wafer cookies, plus 1 for garnish
¼ cup chocolate chips
1 ounce Baileys Irish Cream
1 ounce Kahlúa
1 ounce Godiva chocolate liqueur

Combine the ice cream, the 4 cookies, chocolate chips, Baileys, Kahlúa, and chocolate liqueur in a blender and blend for about 5 seconds. Add about a half cup of ice and blend until smooth. Pour into a tall cocktail glass and garnish with the remaining wafer cookie.

85 JAVA SHERRY CHIP

Sherry added to chocolate, coffee, or cream is a match made in heaven—once you've tried using it in this way, you'll want to use it all the time.

1 large scoop vanilla ice cream
¼ cup chocolate chips
Shot of coffee (or espresso)
1 ounce sherry (you can use a cream sherry that is a little sweeter, if preferred)
1 ounce Kahlúa
3 coffee beans, for garnish

Combine the ice cream, chocolate chips, coffee, sherry, and Kahlúa in a blender and blend for about 5 seconds. Add about 1 cup of ice and blend until smooth. Pour into a tall cocktail glass and garnish with the coffee beans.

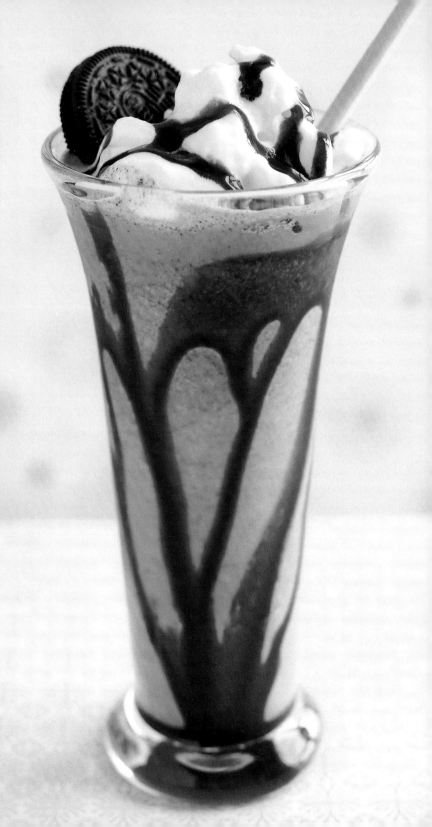

86 FROZEN OREO COOKIE

Chocolate syrup
1 large scoop vanilla ice cream
4 Oreo cookies, plus 1 for garnish
1 ounce Baileys Irish Cream
1 ounce Godiva chocolate liqueur
Whipped cream, for garnish

Swirl the chocolate syrup around the sides of a Hurricane glass or
other tall glass. Combine the ice cream, the 4 Oreos, Baileys, and
chocolate liqueur in a blender and blend for about 5 seconds. Add a
few cubes of ice and blend until smooth. Pour into the swirled glass
and garnish with whipped cream, more chocolate syrup, and the
remaining Oreo.

87 FROZEN CHOCOLATE FONDUE

MAKES 2 SERVINGS

1 ounce cognac
½ ounce Frangelico
½ ounce Godiva chocolate liqueur
2 tablespoons Nutella
1 large scoop vanilla ice cream
Milk, if needed
Sliced fruit and berries of your choice, for serving

Combine the cognac, Frangelico, chocolate liqueur, Nutella, and
ice cream in a blender and blend for about 5 seconds. Add about
1 cup of ice and blend until smooth. (If the mixture is too thick in
the blender, add a little milk to thin it.) Pour into two small cocktail
glasses. Serve with sliced fruit and berries.

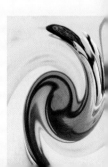

88 CHERRY VANILLA CRÈME

1 large scoop vanilla ice cream
1 ounce vanilla vodka
½ ounce Cherry Heering
1 tablespoon black cherry marmalade
Ground nutmeg, for garnish

Combine the ice cream, vodka, Cherry Heering, and marmalade in a blender and blend for about 5 seconds. Add about 1 cup of ice and blend until smooth. Pour into a cocktail glass and garnish with nutmeg.

89 STRAWBERRY SHORTCAKE

1 large scoop vanilla ice cream
3 strawberries
1 ounce vanilla vodka
Strawberry and piece of fluffy white cake, for garnish

Combine the ice cream, strawberries, and vodka in a blender and blend for about 5 seconds. Add about a half cup of ice and blend until smooth. Pour into a cocktail glass. Garnish with the strawberry and the piece of cake on the rim of the glass.

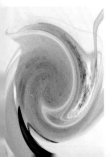

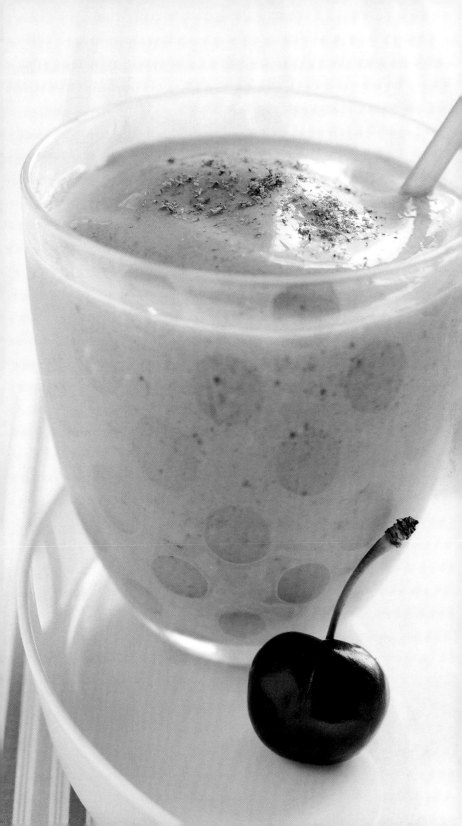

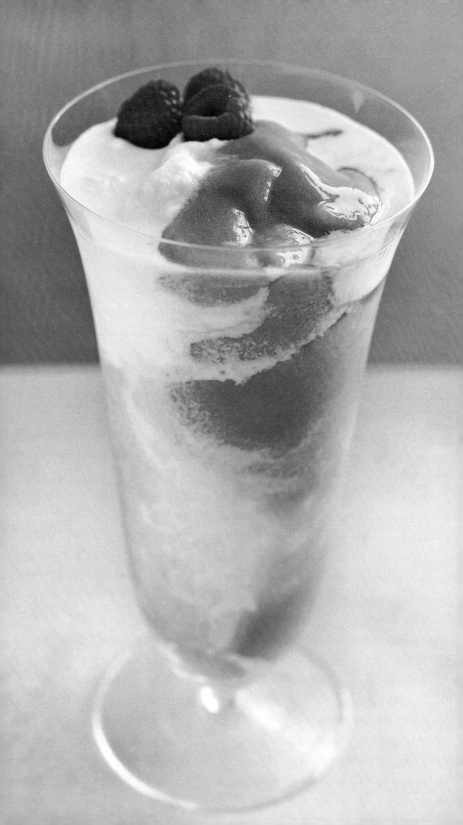

90 WHITE CHOCOLATE RASPBERRY TRIFLE

This is a visually fun cocktail. It takes a little more time because you need to blend the components separately in two different blender cups. If desired, top with fresh berries.

BLENDER CUP 1:
- 1 scoop vanilla ice cream
- 1½ ounces white crème de cacao
- 1 ounce light cream

BLENDER CUP 2:
- 1 scoop raspberry sorbet
- 1 ounce raspberry liqueur (such as Mathilde)
- 1 ounce orange juice

Combine the ice cream, crème de cacao, and light cream in a blender cup and blend for about 5 seconds. Add a few cubes of ice and blend until smooth. Then combine the sorbet, raspberry liqueur, and orange juice in another blender cup and blend for about 5 seconds. Add a few cubes of ice and blend until smooth. Pour the contents from both cups at the same time into a tall glass such as a Hurricane glass. The two mixtures will blend together, but still be separate in the glass, for an interesting two-color look.

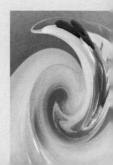

91 FROZEN GRASSHOPPER

1 large scoop mint chocolate chip ice cream
1½ ounces green crème de menthe
1½ ounces white crème de cacao
Mint sprig, for garnish

Combine the ice cream, crème de menthe, and crème de cacao in a
blender and blend for about 5 seconds. Add about a half cup of ice
and blend until smooth. Pour into a cocktail glass and garnish with
the mint sprig.

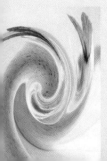

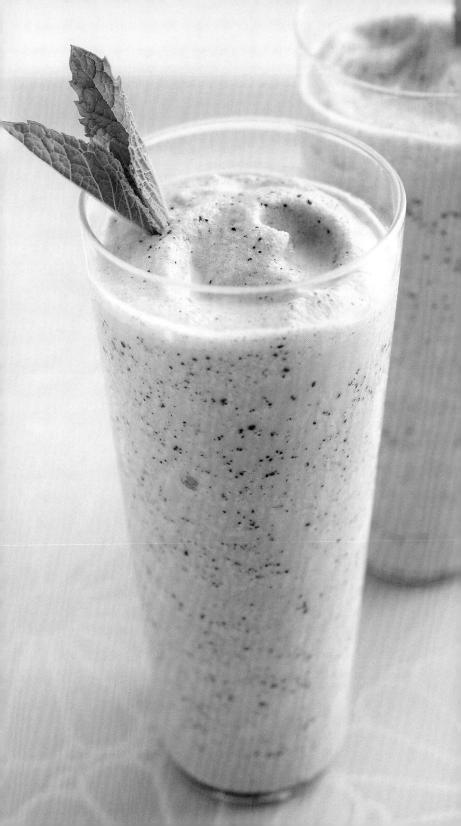

92 COOL CARAMEL FLAN

4 ounces milk or light cream
1 egg yolk
1 ounce Navan vanilla liqueur
1 ounce sweetened condensed milk
½ ounce Frangelico
1 teaspoon raw sugar (turbinado sugar), plus extra for garnish
Caramel sauce, for garnish

Combine the milk, egg yolk, vanilla liqueur, condensed milk,
Frangelico, and sugar in a blender and blend for about 5 seconds.
Add about 1 cup of ice and blend until smooth. Pour into a cocktail
glass and garnish with a sprinkle of sugar and a swirl of caramel
sauce on the top of the drink.

93 BOURBON APPLE SLUSH

1 green apple, peeled, cored, and sliced
1 ounce water
2 teaspoons raw sugar (turbinado sugar)
Dash of ground cinnamon
Dash of ground nutmeg, plus extra for garnish
½ vanilla bean
1½ ounces bourbon

In a sauté pan over medium heat, sauté the apples with the water, sugar, cinnamon, nutmeg, and vanilla bean. Keep stirring until the apples have softened and caramelized, 5 to 7 minutes, adding more water if needed. Let cool. Pour into a blender and blend for about 5 seconds. Add about a half cup of ice and the bourbon and blend until smooth. Pour into a cocktail glass and garnish with nutmeg.

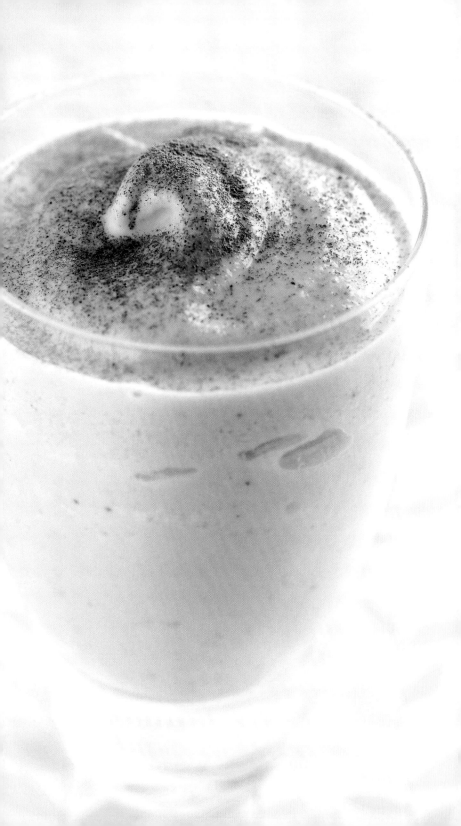

94 BANGKOK BANANA FREEZE

½ banana, peeled
2 to 3 ounces light cream or milk
1½ ounces reposado tequila
1 ounce sweetened condensed milk
½ teaspoon sweetened cocoa powder, plus extra for garnish
¼ teaspoon curry powder
¼ teaspoon ground cardamom, plus extra for garnish

Combine the banana, cream, tequila, condensed milk, cocoa powder, curry, and cardamom in a blender and blend for about 5 seconds. Add about a half cup of ice and blend until smooth. Pour into a cocktail glass and garnish with a sprinkle of ground cardamom and cocoa.

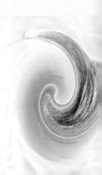

95 MOCHA FLIP

1 large scoop coffee ice cream
1 egg yolk
1 ounce Kahlúa
1 ounce dark crème de cacao
Coffee beans, for garnish

Combine the ice cream, egg yolk, Kahlúa, and crème de cacao in
a blender and blend for about 5 seconds. Add about 1 cup of ice
and blend until smooth. Pour into a cocktail glass and garnish with
coffee beans.

96 PUMPKIN JACK

2 ounces light cream or milk
1½ ounces pumpkin puree (from a can)
1½ ounces sweetened condensed milk
1½ ounces spiced rum
¾ ounce Hiram Walker pumpkin spice liqueur
Dash of ground cinnamon
Dash of ground nutmeg, plus extra for garnish
Whipped cream, for garnish (optional)

Combine the cream, pumpkin puree, condensed milk, spiced rum,
pumpkin spice liqueur, cinnamon, and nutmeg in a blender and
blend for about 5 seconds. Add about a half cup of ice and blend
until smooth. Pour into a cocktail glass. Garnish with a dash of
nutmeg and a dollop of whipped cream, if desired.

97 MATAHORN

1 scoop coconut sorbet
2 ounces light cream or milk
1 ounce coconut rum
1 ounce dark rum
½ ounce coconut cream (such as Coco Lopez)
1 teaspoon sweetened grated coconut, plus extra for garnish

Combine the sorbet, light cream, coconut rum, dark rum, coconut cream, and grated coconut in a blender and blend for about 5 seconds. Add about 1 cup of ice and blend until smooth. Pour into a cocktail glass and garnish with grated coconut.

98 FROZEN PB & J

1 scoop vanilla ice cream
½ banana, peeled (optional)
4 raspberries
1 ounce Frangelico
1 ounce Chambord
2 tablespoons creamy peanut butter
Toast point spread with peanut butter and jelly, for garnish

Combine the ice cream, banana, if desired, raspberries, Frangelico,
Chambord, and peanut butter in a blender and blend for about
5 seconds. Add about a half cup of ice and blend until smooth. Pour
into a cocktail glass. Garnish with the toast point.

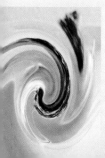

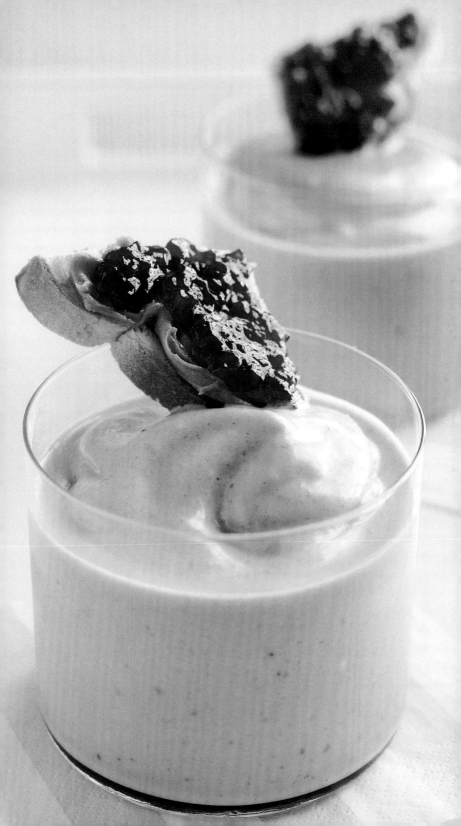

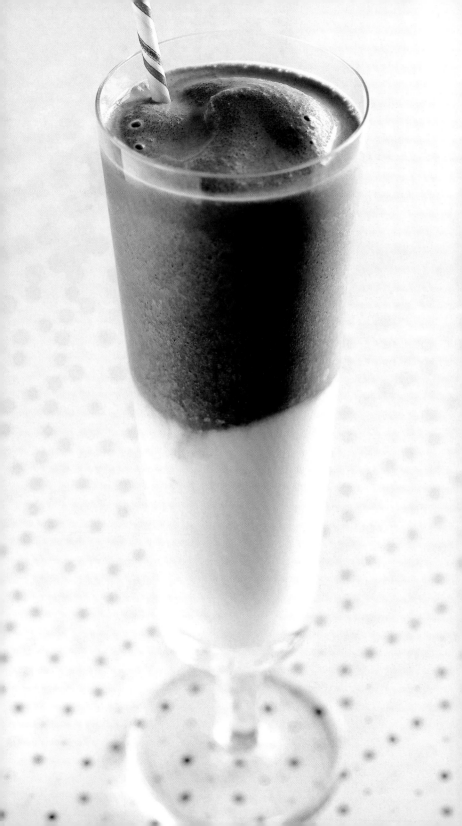

99 PENGUIN

This cocktail is a duo-layer drink that is fun to serve.

BLENDER CUP 1:
    1 scoop vanilla ice cream
    1½ ounces Navan vanilla liqueur

BLENDER CUP 2:
    1 scoop chocolate ice cream
    1 ounce dark crème de cacao
    1 ounce Baileys mint chocolate liqueur
    Chocolate syrup

Combine the vanilla ice cream and vanilla liqueur in a blender cup and blend for about 5 seconds. Add a few cubes of ice and blend until smooth. Set aside. Combine the chocolate ice cream, crème de cacao, and Baileys in another blender cup and blend for about 5 seconds. Add a few cubes of ice and blend until smooth. (The contents of Blender Cup 1 should be much thicker than those of Blender Cup 2.) Pour the contents of Blender Cup 1 into a tall glass such as a Hurricane glass. Pour the contents of Blender Cup 2 on top. It should remain layered for a black-and-white drink.

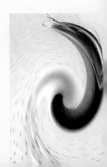

100 FROZEN HOT CHOCOLATE

Inspired by the classic drink served at Serendipity in New York City. The key to this drink is making real homemade hot chocolate. It's hard to duplicate that cooked, caramelized quality without actually making it from scratch. The other key to this recipe is to let the hot chocolate chill completely before blending it; otherwise it will melt the ice rapidly and you'll be left with watered-down cold chocolate milk.

1 cup milk
2 tablespoons sugar
1 ounce water
1 tablespoon unsweetened cocoa powder
¼ teaspoon vanilla extract
1½ ounces Godiva chocolate liqueur
3 mini marshmallows, for garnish
Gourmet chocolate pieces, for garnish (optional)

In a saucepan over medium heat, combine the milk, sugar, water, cocoa powder, and vanilla. Stir constantly until it starts to boil. Place in the refrigerator until completely cooled.

Combine the cooled hot chocolate and chocolate liqueur in a blender with 4 ice cubes. Blend until smooth. (Add and blend in additional sugar, if needed.) Pour into a cocktail glass. Garnish with the mini marshmallows and chocolate pieces, if desired.

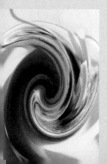

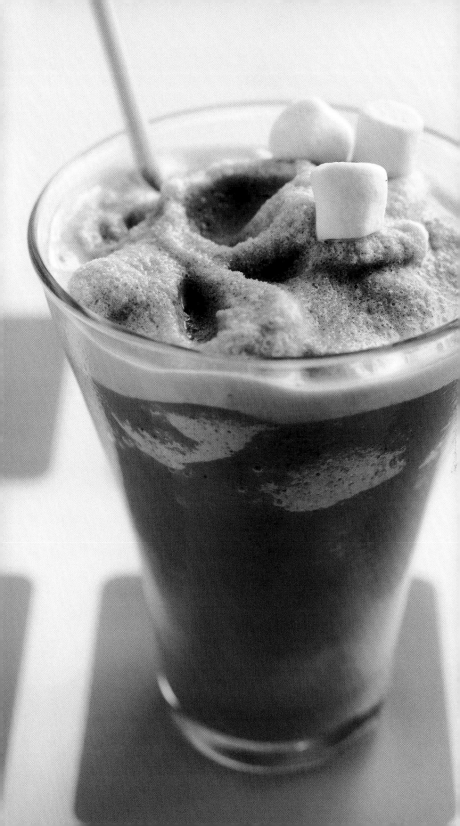

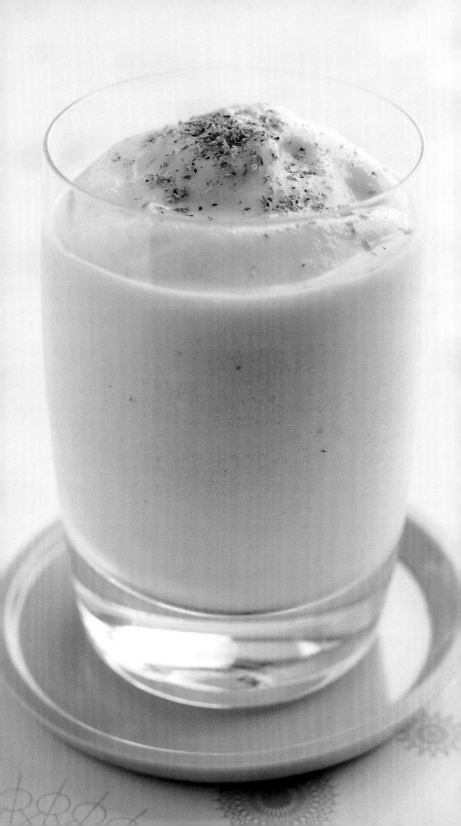

101 FROZEN NOG

1 scoop French vanilla ice cream
1 egg yolk
¾ ounce spiced rum
¾ ounce brandy
Dash of ground nutmeg, plus extra for garnish
3 drops of vanilla extract

Combine the ice cream, egg yolk, rum, brandy, nutmeg, and vanilla in a blender and blend for about 5 seconds. Add about a half cup of ice and blend until smooth. Pour into a small cocktail glass and garnish with nutmeg.

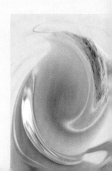

index